MATERIAL BELIEFS
INTERACTION RESEARCH STUDIO

GW00632234

MATERIAL BELIEFS
Interaction Research Studio

This publication marks the end of EPSRC grant EP/E035051/1 – 'Material Beliefs: Collaborations for Public Engagement Between Engineers and Designers'

Edited by Jacob Beaver, Tobie Kerridge and Sarah Pennington
Designed by Hyperkit
Printed by Lecturis

First published in Great Britain 2009 by Goldsmiths, University of London, New Cross, London SE14 6NW

Additional copies of this publication are available from: Interaction Research Studio, Department of Design, Goldsmiths, University of London, New Cross, London SE14 6NW

ISBN 978-1-904158-95-0

This publication has been supported by the EPSRC

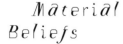
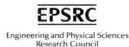

Engineering and Physical Sciences Research Council

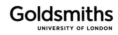

UNIVERSITY OF LONDON

ABOUT THIS BOOK

Material Beliefs was a two-year research project, based at the Interaction Research Studio in the Department of Design at Goldsmiths, University of London, and funded by the Engineering and Physical Sciences Research Council. The project brought together a network of designers, engineers, scientists and social scientists to explore potential implications of emerging biomedical and cybernetic technologies. The ambition was to produce prototypes, exhibitions and debates that would move scientific research out of laboratories into public spaces.

Four designers facilitated the work. They developed relationships with biomedical and cybernetic researchers at UK labs and institutes, guiding a design process in which unfinished scientific research became embodied in speculative products. By responding to social and cultural questions about our expectations of emerging technology, these productions acted as suggestions, not for potential products, but for alternative and often provocative roles for biotechnology in everyday life.

From the outset there was a commitment to involve others in this process, as it developed, and as much as possible. We invited students and young people into the labs, and took work in progress to museums. Researchers became visiting tutors in design departments, patients became expert advisers to researchers, students challenged complex research, and biomedicine was discussed in galleries. It was confusing and exhilarating. As a result of the diversity of this expanded network of people, institutional boundaries became challenged by conversations between individuals.

Not everything happened as we intended, not least because of the range of expectations inherent in such a large and diverse group. But surprises are often the best part of research projects like this. The aim of this book is not only to show the development of the prototypes, and the debates they engendered about science and society at public events, but also to give voice to the conversations that both propelled and challenged the project.

In drawing together the activities of that two-year period, the publication of this book also marks the point when many of those involved are looking towards future activities. Keep an eye on the website, and get in touch if there is something you want to talk about.

www.materialbeliefs.com
info@materialbeliefs.com

ACKNOWLEDGEMENTS

Project leader
TOBIE KERRIDGE

Principal investigator
BILL GAVER

Collaboration leaders
ELIO CACCAVALE, JIMMY LOIZEAU,
SUSANA SOARES

Project manager
ANDY ROBINSON

Evaluation
SAVITA CUSTEAD, EMILY DAWSON

Advisory group
ANTHONY DUNNE, MIKE MICHAEL,
LESLEY PATERSON, FIONA RABY,
NOEL SHARKY

Project mentor
RAY MATHIAS

EPSRC
JOANNA COLEMAN, KATE MILLER

Publication
JACOB BEAVER, SARAH
PENNINGTON

Documentary film and DVD
STEVE JACKMAN, DANIEL
OSKIEWICZ

**Identity, website and
publication design**
HYPERKIT

Website development
KESTER HYNDS

**Carnivorous Domestic
Entertainment Robots**
JAMES AUGER, TREVOR HARVEY,
IOANNIS IEROPOULOS, TOMMASO
LANZA, CHRIS MELHUISH, JULIAN
VINCENT, ALAN WINFIELD,
ALEKSANDAR ZIVANOVIC

Neuroscope
PAUL DORE, JULIA DOWNES,
MARK HAMMOND, DAVID MUTH,
SLAWOMIR NASUTO, KEVIN
WARWICK, BEN WHALLEY,
DIMITRIS XYDAS

Vital Signs
ANDY BOUCHER, TONY CASS,
REVITAL COHEN, TIMOTHY
CONSTANDINOU, JAYDEN DESIR,
NATASJA DESIR, PANTELIS
GEORGIOU, OLIVE MURPHY, ROS
OAKLEY, NICK OLIVER, DAVID
NOONAN, RAY THOMPSON, CHRIS
TOUMAZOU

Bonsai Cells
JULIE DANIELS, DIANNE FORD,
AUBREY DE GREY, ANNA HARRIS,
CHRIS MASON, ANDERS SANDBERG,
LUISA WAKELING

Interviewees
ADRIAN BOWER, BEN HANSON,
JOANNE INGRAM, CLAIRE ROCKS,
PETER WALTER

Collaboration workshop
STEVE BENFORD, KAREN CHAM,
JO COLEMAN, TOM HULBERT,
VICKY JONES, SARAH KETLEY,
ZOE LAUGHLIN, MARK PALMER,
JANE PROPHET, PETE SAMPSON,
NICOLA TRISCOTT, IAN THOMPSON,
BRENDAN WALKER

Goldsmiths
THOMAS ADAMS, LYNDA AGILI,
JULIEN ANDERSON, JOHN BOWERS,
MARTIN CONREEN, JUSTIN DAVIN-
SMITH, RUTH EDWARDS-GRACE,
MARIE FALLON, PETE GRAVER,
ROSARIO HURTADO, NADINE
JARVIS, PIPPA KRISHNAN, ANA
LISA, CATHERINE MCGEOGHEGAN,
UNA QUIN, ANN SCHLACHTER,
MATT WARD, ANDREW
WEATHERHEAD, ALEX WILKIE

Events
CATERINA ALBANO, MARY
ARBER, SHAHID AZIZ, OLIVER
BANCROFT, IVANA BAGO, JAMES
BELL, NELLY BEN HAYOUN, WILL
CAREY, ANDREW CHETTY, PATRICK
DEGENAAR, AMIR EFTEKHAR,
ROB FENTON, ROBERTO FEO, DAISY
GINSBERG, RICK HALL, CLAIRE
HARRISON, VEDA HARRISON, JULLIE
HILL, ROWAN JURY, CATHRINE
KRAMER, BRIGITTE LELIEVRE, OLGA
MAJCEN, TOBIN MAY, ANDY MIAH,
KOSTIS MICHELAKIS, SUNCICA
OSTOJC, LUCINDA PARISH, WANDA
PILIPKIEWICZ, SASCHA POHFLEPP,
DOMINIQUE RENN, SABINE
SEYMOUR, LAURA SILLARS, NAOMI
TEMPLE, JOHN WILLIAMS, IZABELA
WOJCICKA, JENNIFER WONG,
SIMON WOODS

CONTENTS

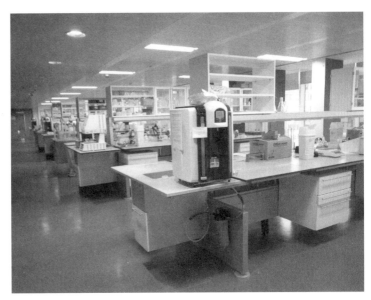

Fig. 0.1

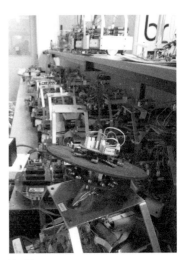

Fig. 0.2

Material Beliefs was a research project based at Goldsmiths, University of London, which explored two pressing questions of our time. In this age of incipient bioengineering, are we becoming in some way products of our own technologies? How do we, the general public, relate to the engineers and scientists behind these technologies, and how do they relate to us?

Many interested parties, in industry and government and the media, have something to say about these questions, prompted by concerns about healthcare, economics, ethics and religion. But what does the general public say? And who is the general public? Back in the 1950s, C.P. Snow made a famous distinction between the 'two cultures' of science and art, ever at loggerheads. Nowadays a more useful distinction might be made between specialists and non-specialists. The modern world is full of specialists, in government and industry, in the media and everywhere else, and yet all these people are non-specialists outside their particular field of expertise. (A biotechnologist, for example, is a non-specialist when it comes to biomechanics or tissue engineering.) This is where design comes in.

The inspiration for this project came from the perception that the discipline of design, and more specifically the tactics employed in certain design research, might act on the many issues surrounding bioengineering technologies and public engagement as an integrating and illuminating force, by bringing very different people together and provoking debate. Design, especially interaction design, lies somewhere between the sciences and the humanities (depending on who you talk

0.1 *Wet lab, Institute of Biomedical Engineering*
0.2 *Robot stack, Bristol Robotics Lab*

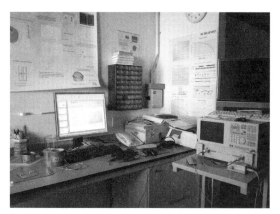

Fig. 0.3

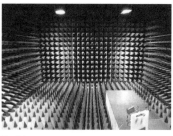

Fig. 0.4

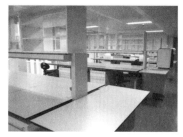

Fig. 0.5

0.3 *Electronics lab, Institute of*
Biomedical Engineering
0.4 *Anechoic chamber, Institute of*
Biomedical Engineering
0.5 *Wet lab, Institute of Biomedical*
Engineering

to), as it is concerned with both the products of digital technology and the implications of those products for all of us, including their creators. (Cybernetics engineers may be hidden from public view in their labs, but when they use a mobile phone they are as much – or as little – a product of the technology as other users.) Could design's unique position be utilised to open up a new space of communication which crosses the increasingly blurred boundaries between 'the expert' and 'the public', and between our bodies and the technological systems we inhabit? To put this more simply: might the material – the tangible products – that emerge from research combining design and engineering, throw some light on our beliefs about ourselves, and our future selves?

Material Beliefs was, by definition, a collaborative endeavour. The parties involved – principally biomedical engineers and 'speculative' designers, but also social scientists, doctors, school children and many others – were as varied as the issues touched upon. This had two main consequences. First, strategic questions were paramount: what role does each party play, and what do they expect to get out of it? Second, the process was as important as the results, and as open to question. Indeed, you could say that the most telling results were the questions which arose at each stage of the process, from the initial meetings between designers and engineers to their reflections months later.

This book represents an attempt to gather together all those questions, informing them with as much context as possible, and offering them in a way which captures as closely as possible the manner in which they arose. Images of 'carnivorous' robots rub shoulders with observations by sociologists, insights into cutting-edge biomedicine, policy documents about public perceptions of engineering, and a child's drawing of a cyborg. Structure is provided by chronology: the book runs from the first stirrings of the project in July 2006 (a grant application to the Engineering and Physical Sciences Research Council) to its ending in December 2008, when focus groups, involving some of the key players, discussed the rewards and disappointments of Material Beliefs. The chronology is framed by two essays, by Mike Michael and Emily Dawson, and an interview with Tony Dunne, which offer perspectives on different aspects of the project. Other voices are heard throughout the book, typically at the beginning of each section, where remarks by different collaborators highlight some of the themes that emerged.

A DVD is attached to the back of the book, containing short films of some of the public events in which Material Beliefs participated, and interviews with designers and engineers who worked on, or influenced, the project.

JACOB BEAVER
April 2009

Chapter 1

PIPE LAGGERS AND BIONIC EYES

—

SCOPING THE PROJECT

1.0

PIPE LAGGERS
AND BIONIC EYES
—
SCOPING
THE PROJECT

> 'The term "engineer" isn't particularly well thought of. So your "thermal engineer" may actually turn out to be a pipe lagger.'
> CHRIS MELHUISH
> *Bristol Robotics Laboratory*
>
> 'Are bionic eyes possible? We believe so.'
> PATRICK DEGENAAR
> *Institute of Biomedical Engineering, Imperial College London*

Recent reports by the Engineering Technology Board (ETB) and other engineering bodies have spoken of a 'crisis' in engineering. The proportion of undergraduate students is down; skilled technicians are dwindling. Why isn't engineering seen as 'sexy' at a time when nanotechnology and silicon technology are drawing close enough (almost) to begin fulfilling the sci-fi fantasies of the past 50 years? Is it because 'the more developed a country is, the less relevant engineering seems as a career, and therefore the less inspiring'? [1]

Whatever the reason, the *impact* of scientific and engineering research, particularly in the field of biomedicine, is starting to show. Consider stem cell therapy for eye diseases, cochlea implants for the deaf, the increasing use of digital insulin pumps for diabetics. Whether or not people want to study engineering, they ought to care about its creations and, ideally, have a voice in their development – or so thinks the Engineering and Physical Sciences Research Council (EPSRC), which runs a Public Engagement Programme. It was this programme that granted funds to Material Beliefs in 2007, providing for a two-year project in which designers and engineers were to collaborate in unforeseeable ways.

The project began slowly, tentatively. The small team at Goldsmiths made contact first with other design researchers, and then with research engineers involved, in one way or another, with biology or medicine. The designers interviewed the engineers, on film, simply to see what – if anything – came out of the experience. We knew that we wanted to make the scientists' labs 'permeable', but we didn't know how (apart from theoretical notions about 'design-led processes' focusing on 'everyday situations'). We knew that 'the public' needed to be 'engaged', but we didn't have a clear idea of who exactly the public were, or why 'they' might want to engage. On top of all that, we had no idea how the 'shared practices' of engineers and designers might operate, practically or conceptually.

What we did know was that there were many interesting, and potentially interested, people out there ...

[1] An insight from the Human Development Index, as described by Sir Anthony Cleaver, Chairman of the ETB, in a speech he gave in 2008.

1.1

ENGAGING WITH ENGAGEMENT

–

THE COMPLEXITIES OF MATERIAL BELIEFS

Essay by Mike Michael
Centre for the Study of Invention and Social Process
February 2009

My initial reaction to the Material Beliefs brief was one of confusion. Like a lot of people, I suspect, my general response was, 'what is the point' of these collaborations between engineers (of one sort or another) and designers (of one sort or another)? This was an echo of a response to earlier design-oriented public engagements with science and technology, especially that of the Biojewellery project.[1] To recall: the Biojewellery project entailed the donation of bone cells by couples. These cells were taken from the jaw during the removal of wisdom teeth. The cells were subsequently cultured around a ring-shaped bioactive scaffold. This was then made into rings incorporating precious metals, and the rings were exchanged by the couples. The project generated a series of events, and publications and statements were sent out into the world – exhibitions, press releases, web and hard-copy documentation. As far as I can tell, however, only minimal effort was made to gauge the public's response to Biojewellery. Whenever I mentioned this to my colleagues in social science, their reactions were, after an initial 'yuk' response to the very idea of biojewellery, just like mine: 'what was the point of that?' And when I described the projects of Material Beliefs I was again met with similar puzzlement. Despite the claims that this was all 'public engagement', it was unlike any sort of public engagement with which we were familiar. Even so, I did find this designerly approach intriguing, though at first I couldn't understand why. Let me expand.

From one prominent social scientific perspective, public engagement with science is generally about facilitating the expression of lay people's views about

'We like to pitch things at every level – from school children, the general press, the technical press for hobbyists, to the top level, scientific journals. I've deliberately arranged the list in a hierarchy I don't believe in. If I were asked to nominate the one I thought the most important, it would be the thirteen-year-old school children. Clever scientists can look after themselves.'

ADRIAN BOWER
Department of Mechanical Engineering, University of Bath

1.1.1 *Wisdom tooth extraction at Guy's Hospital – Biojewellery project*
1.1.2 *Scaffold, bone sample and prototype ring – Biojewellery project*
1.1.3 *Bonsai Cells exhibited at the Royal Institution*
1.1.4 *Neuroscope exhibited at LABoral*
1.1.5 *CDER exhibited at LABoral*
1.1.6 *Vital Signs exhibited at LABoral*

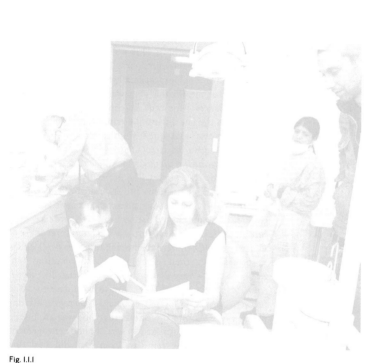

Fig. I.I.I

Fig. I.I.2

this scientific issue or that technological controversy. Numerous techniques – for example, citizens' juries, citizens' panels, consensus conferences, deliberative polling[2] – have been designed to enable publics to speak freely about their concerns, views, understandings, and to directly address these to relevant experts. The aim is to allow public concern to enter democratically into the innovation and science policy process. Needless to say, all this has been criticised on numerous grounds: are these techniques – or what I prefer to call 'formalised mechanisms of voicing'[3] – really enabling the public's voice? How do they actually link up to forms of governance? Do they entail real engagement or are they, in fact, instances of public relations? Is dissent accommodated, or is there an emphasis on consensus that forecloses the more radical forms of scientific citizenship?[4]

In reflecting on the Biojewellery project and, subsequently, on the engagement dimensions of the Material Beliefs projects, I came to realise that the tenets underpinning the social scientific versions of public engagement were being purposely undermined. It was this that made both Biojewellery and Material Beliefs

so disorienting, and yet so enthralling. Here, 'public engagement' did not necessarily imply an imminent, discrete technological problem or an urgent, definable scientific controversy; there seemed to be hardly any system in the gathering and recording of 'public' views; there appeared to be little effort to craft a representative digest of such views, as an aid to policy-making; more broadly, none of the designers seemed overly bothered about the citizenliness of the public, or concerned that they might have a scholarly 'duty' to mediate the democratic process so that the public voice could be better heard in the corridors of power.

This might be a gross simplification of these design projects and the aims underlying them. Nevertheless, it seems to me that there is, from a social scientific perspective, something very odd going on here. As I see it, the difference hinges on a contrasting set of tacit notions about 'the public', 'engagement', and 'science and technology'.

For the designers and managers of Material Beliefs, the public seems to be composed of more or less fully-rounded persons, able more or less to confront with cognitive and

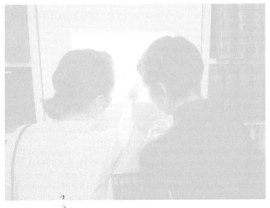

Fig. 1.1.3

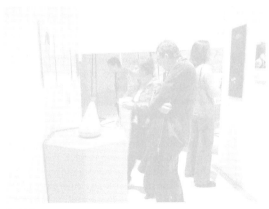

Fig. 1.1.4

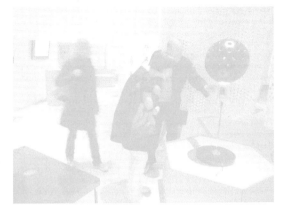

Fig. 1.1.5

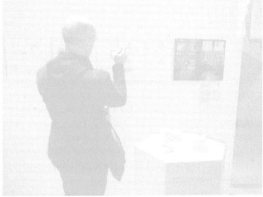

Fig. 1.1.6

emotional maturity (for want of a better phrase) such novel – indeed, strange – designerly artifacts as Caccavale's Neuroscope, or Auger and Loizeau's Carnivorous Domestic Entertainment Robots. What is particularly interesting is that this 'maturity' is characterised by a capacity to entertain, deal with, and explore the confusion, ambiguity, blurriness of the issues embodied in these objects (on which, more below). This is a version of the public that does not suffer from either intellectual or democratic deficit – rather, it is a constituency whose role is not to be 'citizenly' within a context of policy-making, but thoughtful within a context of complexity.

The corollary is that the idea of engagement is very different across social scientific and design disciplines. As I've hinted, for the social scientist, 'engagement' entails a doing of citizenliness in which issues are grasped and clarified, positions are distinguished and demarcated, arguments enunciated and attributed. Of course, there was plenty of this in the engagement activities of Material Beliefs, notably in the *Techno Bodies; Hybrid Life?* event at the Dana Centre in the Science Museum. But it strikes me that 'engagement' also has another array of meanings:

something akin to the 'artistic encounter'. Material Belief's objects are quasi-artistic, and they are meant to evoke in their audiences not so much a need for clarity, but a *desire for complexity*.

This can be put another way. The engagement of social science is ultimately concerned with solutions: decision-making processes in which the voice of the public is properly featured, and which yield policies that address the pressing techno-scientific questions of the day. Here, 'science' and 'society' are brought together to deliberate, but the process of deliberation by and large does not trouble the divide between science and society, expert and lay, or scientist and public. In the 'event' of such engagement, science and society can 'be together'. However, there is an alternative conceptualization of 'event'. Mariam Fraser, drawing on work by Whitehead, Stengers and Deleuze, notes that we can also view the event (in our case, the event of engagement) as a moment where entities (in our case, science and society), rather than simply 'being together', also 'become together'.[5] As such, the event is characterised by a sort of mutual changing. In the process, what emerges is not 'solutions' but better problems; or rather, the event should entail what Fraser calls 'inventive problem-making' – which is an engagement with complexity.[6]

Critical to this process of 'inventive problem-making' is the other key component of the event of engagement, namely the designed objects themselves. This stuff – literally, the stuff of Soares's Bonsai Cells or the digital plasters of Kerridge's Vital Signs – is difficult. It has implications that are good and bad, individual and collective, internal and external, biological and cultural, emancipatory and authoritarian, modest and arrogant, cruel and funny, academic and commercial, serious and playful ... It alludes to cutting-edge science and technology, to hackneyed ideals around health and environment, to science fiction (both utopian and dystopian), to historical narratives of oppression and discovery, to horror and humour. This stuff is, in Donna Haraway's terminology, a black hole.[7] If social scientific forms of engagement regard 'science and technology' in terms of complicated controversy, Material Beliefs suggests a view in which 'science and technology' is hugely more variegated. That is to say, Material Belief's designed artefacts spiral out in many conceptual directions, raising questions about a multitude of indistinct issues surrounding science and technology. And so we turn full circle, back to the different versions of 'the public'. For, rather than encouraging 'the public' in the pursuit of argumentational transparency on a specific set of issues, the artefacts invite a subjective[8] engagement with their puzzling opacity – their black-hole-ness.

Now, key to this opacity is, ironically, the everydayness of these artefacts.[9] They have been designed to sit within the mundane. Once we have got over the novelty of insect-consuming machines, or plasters that update remote databases about our bodily condition, these objects should drift into unnoticeability. We can, perhaps dimly, imagine a time when these artefacts go about their business with the same sort of invisibility as a toaster or the central heating system.[10] What are the implications of this inkling of domesticity? At the very least, there would need to be a change in us. We would have to co-become with the artefacts in order for them to operate seamlessly within our everyday lives. But what would we become? The potential ordinariness of the artefacts – an aspect that is not always apparent in arguments over scientific and technological innovation, where expectations are routinely raised, novelty is emphasised, and hopes and hype mingle in the pursuit of regulatory or commercial advantage[11] – makes us aware that we would have to turn into ... something else. Something uncomfortable, perhaps. We confront our own opacity through these artefacts – or rather, we co-become with them to inventively make problems about what 'we' might become.

1 *Biojewellery* (2007). www.biojewellery.com/project.html (accessed 17 July 2007).

2 See, for example, Cass, N. (2006) Participatory-Deliberative Engagement: A Literature Review. Manchester: School of Environment and Development, Manchester University. www..manchester.ac.uk/sed/research/beyond_nimbyism.

3 Michael, M. & Brown, N. (2005) 'Scientific Citizenships: Self-Representations of Xenotransplantation's Publics', *Science as Culture* 14: 38-57.

4 See, for example, Elam, M. & Bertilsson, M. (2003) 'Consuming, Engaging and Confronting Science: The Emerging Dimensions of Scientific Citizenship', *European Journal of Social Theory* 6: 233-251; Hagendijk, R. & Kallerud, E. (2003) 'Changing Conceptions and Practices of Governance in Science and Technology in Europe: A Framework for Analysis', Discussion Paper Two, Science, Technology and Governance in Europe; Michael, M. (in press) Publics Performing Publics: Of PiGs, PiPs and Politics. Public Understanding of Science.

5 Fraser, M. (forthcoming) 'Facts, Ethics and Event,' in C. Bruun Jensen and K. Rödje (eds) Deleuzian Intersections in Science, Technology and Anthropology. New York: Berghahn Press.

6 This problem-making also folds back on to the analyst of the event, who undergoes a 'transformation of the will' such that, to paraphrase Fraser, both the analyst of, and the participant in, the event are likely to be transformed.

7 'For the complex or boundary objects in which I am interested, the mythic, textual, political, organic and economic dimensions implode. That is, they collapse into each other in a knot of extraordinary density that constitutes the objects themselves. In my sense, storytelling is ... a fraught practice for narrating complexity in such a field of knots or black holes.' (p. 63) Haraway, D. (1994) 'A game of cat's cradle: science studies, feminist theory, cultural studies', *Configurations*, 2, 59-71.

8 'Subjective' is not quite the right term as it presupposes a pre-existing consciousness that does the puzzling. Whitehead's term 'superject' is preferable because it points to the way that such artefacts can come together with people in complex events out of which emerge particular – puzzled – types of subjectivity. See Whitehead, A.N. (1929) *Process and Reality: An Essay in Cosmology.* New York: The Free Press; and Halewood, M. and Michael, M. (2008) 'Being a Sociologist and Becoming a Whiteheadian: Concrescing Methodological Tactics', *Theory, Culture and Society*, 25 (4), 31-56.

9 It is, of course, possible to focus upon the specific biological *content* and related assemblages of these design objects in order to unravel their opacity or black-hole-ness. However, as should be clear, I am for present purposes more interested in the *form* – political, social, material – that these artefacts take.

10 Which is not to say that such everyday objects – as parts of socio-technical assemblages – are not generative of novelty or change. For examples of the productivity of the ordinary, see Michael, M. (2000) *Reconnecting Culture, Technology and Nature: From Society to Heterogeneity.* London: Routledge; Michael, M. (2006). *Technoscience and Everyday Life.* Maidenhead, Berks.:Open University Press/McGraw-Hill.

11 See, for example, Brown, N., Rappert, B., & Webster, A. (2000) *Introducing Contested Futures: From Looking into the Future to Looking at the Future.* In Brown, N. et al (eds) Contested Futures: A Sociology of Prospective Techno-Science. Ashgate, Aldershot, 3-20.

1.2

SCIENCE AND SOCIETY
—
PERCEPTIONS OF ENGINEERING

The following extracts from three documents provide some sense of how Material Beliefs arose. The third report of the House of Lords Select Committee on Science and Technology, published in 2000, offered an influential reconsideration of the relationship between science and society. Then comes an extract from an invitation to an EPSRC workshop, where the proposal for Material Beliefs was written, which gives an example of how funding bodies implement policy. The third piece, an article in Imperial College's *Reporter*, announcing the creation of a Chair in Science and Society, shows how policy recommendations filter down to individual institutions.

'I think that the end result – the headline news – like putting cells into the patient and then getting a better visual outcome, obviously it would be difficult to find somebody that wasn't impressed by that. But the rest of it, the day-to-day stuff, how you grow the cells and all the important things that are needed to get to that end point – we're unsure how interested the public are in that.'

JULIE DANIELS
Institute of Ophthalmology, University College London

'When somebody does scientific research, they should be subject to exactly the same rules of observation as the rest of humanity, and people should be able to say, "oh, that was interesting", or "that was well done", or "that's a load of rubbish".'

ADRIAN BOWER
Department of Mechanical Engineering, University of Bath

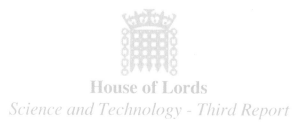

House of Lords
Science and Technology - Third Report

A new mood for dialogue

3.9 Despite all this activity and commitment, we have been told from several quarters that the expression "public understanding of science" may not be the most appropriate label. Sir Robert May called it a "rather backward-looking vision" (Q 28). It is argued that the words imply a condescending assumption that any difficulties in the relationship between science and society are due entirely to ignorance and misunderstanding on the part of the public; and that, with enough public-understanding activity, the public can be brought to greater knowledge, whereupon all will be well. This approach[27] is felt by many of our witnesses to be inadequate; the British Council went so far as to call it "outmoded and potentially disastrous" (p 140).

3.10 As we argued in Chapter 1 above, science cannot ignore its social context. In Chapter 2 we reviewed evidence of a decline in trust; rebuilding trust will require improved communication in both directions. Professor Conway put it thus to the directors of Monsanto, in the context of GM crops: "There is a great deal of talking going on—much of it very emotional and acrimonious. Yet there is very little accountability or transparency in these discussions. The dialogue needs to be better informed, better structured and more inclusive. There may be an opportunity to help create a public space for conversation—to turn down the decibel level and increase the amount of real information and exchange that could lead to a more positive outcome". Or, as Sir Aaron Klug put it[28], "Engagement with society is a two-way process, involving dialogue between different (though not necessarily opposing) sets of values".

3.11 It is therefore increasingly important that non-experts should be able to understand aspects of science and technology which touch their lives. It is also increasingly important that scientists should seek to understand the impact of their work and its possible applications on society and public opinion, not least through the media. They should see themselves as "civic scientists" - a phrase coined by Dr Neal Lane, the US President's Assistant for Science and Technology, whom we were pleased to meet in Washington—that is, as scientists "concerned not just with intriguing intellectual questions but also with using science to help address societal needs"[29]. The new spirit of accountability and the new mood for dialogue are not confined to the United Kingdom, but are being felt equally in the USA.

3.12 In the rest of this chapter we review some of the institutions and activities which currently operate under the term "public understanding of science". As will be seen, many of them are already beginning to respond to the current mood for dialogue between society and science. In Chapter 5 we consider ways to take this dialogue a step further.

27 Referred to in academic parlance as the "deficit model". Back
28 Royal Society Anniversary Address 1999. Back
29 Dr Lane speaking on 29 September 1999. Back

Engineering and Physical Sciences
Research Council

Engineering Ideas in Public Engagement
Call for Participants

Dates: Tuesday 28 – Friday 31 March 2006
Wednesday 3 May – Friday 5 May 2006

Venue: Shrigley Hall, Pott Shrigley, near Macclesfield

Closing date for applications: Midday, Friday 10 February 2006

Thinking Outside the Box

Much has been done and continues to be done in the area of public engagement by scientists, engineers and others about science and engineering; much tried and much learnt with varying degrees of success. With some notable exceptions the majority of effort in public engagement over the last 20 years has addressed science subjects and, to a degree, involved practising scientists, as opposed to engineering. Are there issues in public engagement that pertain particularly to engineering or do we just cut and paste ideas from science engagement? Surely the very nature of engineering demands a fresh analysis even if some of the guiding principles turn out to be similar? Could more be achieved with some concerted thought and funding? What innovative approaches can we find that will enable new thinking between the disparate players involved? Where can we enhance success and build and how and where should we innovate? How do we reach a universal commitment to public engagement by the engineering community – one that recognises that public engagement is integral to the process of engineering and not a quick fix? How do we achieve a step-change in the attitudes of engineers towards public engagement?

An Engineering IDEAS Factory

The concept of an IDEAS Factory is to organise interactive workshops on particular topics, involving 20-30 participants. The focus for this Factory is to explore novel approaches to public engagement and engineering. Some unusual approaches will be tried to encourage participants to contribute as fulsomely as possible. Expect the unexpected!

In addition to the grant schemes already offered by EPSRC for public engagement work, a further, substantial provisional budget has been allocated to fund public engagement in engineering to be taken up by novel and adventurous approaches to these issues.

Fig. I.2.2 *Engineering Ideas in Public Engagement: Call for Participants*

Science and society role for Robert Winston

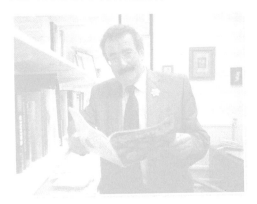

Lord Winston has taken up a role as Professor of Science and Society at Imperial. The freshly created Chair will focus on developing paths for better engagement between scientists and the public through a range of initiatives.

Professor Winston's programme over the next five years will include conducting research into the most effective methods of science engagement and evaluating its impact.

He said: **"The science we do is largely owned by the public and all members of society should feel they are a part of what we do. As scientists, we need to be much more open about the nature of science and its limitations and more engaged with the ethical impact that our work may have."**

Finding methods to ensure that scientists communicate effectively with the public will be a key focus, with the aim of further embedding science communication techniques in Imperial's teaching. He explains: "It is vital for scientists to be able to talk about our research. We need to encourage more students to recognise the importance of this and be able to talk about their work to make it relevant to as many people as possible. This will also have the benefit of stimulating thinking about the impact of scientific work on society in general."

The role will also include helping to expand Imperial's wide range of outreach activities, establishing a dedicated schools laboratory and seminar facility based at the College to give pupils and teachers experience of hands-on science in areas such as DNA analysis and robotics. He adds: "Giving young people the chance to get involved in practical work in a scientific environment is the key to inspiring them to see science as exciting."

Welcoming Lord Winston's appointment to the new Chair, Rector Sir Richard Sykes said: "Robert Winston is one of the UK's most prominent scientists and has an impressive track record of drawing a diverse cross-section of society into scientific conversations. I'm delighted that he will continue this vital work at Imperial."

In addition to his new role as the Chair in Science and Society, Lord Winston will retain his Emeritus Professorship of Fertility Studies at the College.

—Abigail Smith, Communications

£8.9 million award boosts heart research

Finding innovative ways to prevent, diagnose and treat heart and circulatory disease is the focus of a new Centre of Research Excellence at Imperial, established this month through an £8.9 million award from the British Heart Foundation (BHF).

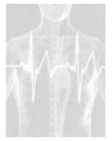

Medical researchers, scientists and engineers from 20 different disciplines at Imperial will join forces in the new Centre. Imperial's clinical researchers will trial new therapies for heart disease and collaborate with geneticists and cell biologists, who are exploring the genes involved in heart disease. Geneticists will team up with computer scientists to analyse the wealth of new data available and biochemists will collaborate with engineers studying the mechanics of blood flow, to design new ways to diagnose and treat heart disease.

The six-year award will support new interdisciplinary research and training programmes, including a PhD training programme for 27 engineers, medical students and bioscientists. The College will also be recruiting 14 postdoctoral fellows and eight specialist registrars.

The BHF hopes that within the lifetime of the award, highly trained researchers will leave the Centre to establish new research groups focusing on heart disease.

Professor Michael Schneider, Director of the new Centre and Head of Cardiovascular Science, said: "I am ecstatic about the award. At Imperial, the BHF Centre can be described best as a triangular alliance among cardiovascular medicine, the underpinning biomedical sciences like genetics and stem cell biology, and leading edge research in the physical sciences such as chemical biology, computational biology and bioengineering."

Professor Peter Weissberg, Medical Director at the BHF, added: "Many of the advances in the prevention, diagnosis and treatment of cardiovascular disease available today are the result of past research undertaken in the UK. The BHF Centres of Research Excellence will ensure that the UK retains its world leading edge and that UK patients are the first to benefit. This investment will create a new generation of world class researchers to lead the fight against heart disease over the coming decades."

—Laura Gallagher, Communications

• The April magazine podcast features an interview with Professor Schneider: www.imperial.ac.uk/media/podcasts

Fig. 1.2.3 *Reporter, the newspaper of Imperial College London*

1.3

EPSRC
PROPOSAL

The next two pages reproduce the funding proposal for Material Beliefs, which was submitted to the EPSRC in July 2006, following the Engineering Ideas workshop. The proposal includes some details about the aims and objectives of the project, and also a description of intended audiences.

'In any research position, it helps your funding profile to do public engagement.'

EMILY DAWSON
Department of Education and Professional Studies, King's College London

'The public engagement section of grant proposals – a lot of people don't have anything to put in that box. You make up a load of waffle about open-door policy in your lab or something like that. But these are tangible things we've done to engage the public with our work, and yeah, I would say that largely it's been an extremely positive experience.'

BEN WHALLEY
The University of Reading, School of Pharmacy

EPSRC
Polaris House, North Star Avenue, Swindon, Wiltshire, United Kingdom SN2 1ET
Telephone +44 (0) 1793 444000
Web http://www.epsrc.ac.uk/

Je-SRP1(EPSRC)
v1.3

COMPLIANCE WITH THE DATA PROTECTION ACT 1998

In accordance with the Data Protection Act 1998, the personal data provided on this form will be processed by EPSRC, and may be held on computerised database and/or manual files. Further details may be found in the **guidance notes**

Standard PROPOSAL

Document Status: WithCouncil

EPSRCReference: EP/E035051/1

Organisation where the Grant would be held

Organisation	Goldsmiths College	Research Organisation Reference:	Kerridge
Division or Department	Design		

Project Title [up to 150 chars]

Material Beliefs - Collaborations for Public Engagement Between Engineers and Designers

Start Date and Duration

a. Proposed start date: 01 October 2006

b. Duration of the grant (months): 24

Applicants

Role	Name	Organisation	Division or Department	How many hours a week will the investigator work on the project?
Principal Investigator	Professor William Gaver	Goldsmiths College	Design	1
Researcher-Co-Investigator	Mr Tobie Kerridge	Goldsmiths College	Design	15

Objectives

List the main objectives of the proposed research in order of priority [up to 4000 chars]

The objective of this proposal is to pair experienced research engineers and designers through a residency program, leading to a series of public exhibitions and engagement events. These events will open up a reflective and critical space around the role of future technology, where the engineers' research can be represented to the public in a stimulating way. There are three core aims:

1.To provide engineers with an expanded and invigorated sense of value in their own research activity.

2.To challenge the working methods of designers by broadening their engagement with engineering processes.

3.To create a range of deliverables that provide a broad audience with a rich set of insights into the potential of engineering research

The third aim is crucial, and the proposal draws on considerable experience of using design as a tool to garner attention, drive debate and provoke independent thought. The proposal is primarily aimed at resourcing a collaborative and reflective space for the development of outputs for public engagement. The precise nature of the tangible outcomes is not predefined; the form, content and themes of the outputs come out of this reflection and subsequent development.

Fig. 1.3.1 *Material Beliefs proposal to EPSRC (page 1)*

Despite this, the proposal takes a strategic view on how best to promote and show these outcomes, by building partnerships with journalists, exhibition venues, conference organisers, institutions and other professionals from the outset. As the form and tone of the outputs become refined, there will be a clear framework for engagement in place. The need for an innovative approach to exhibition is a core concern. This proposal is committed to a thorough analysis of comparable, past events, and looks forward to experimenting with fresh formats by reconsidering how and where the work is shown.

Summary

Describe the proposed research in simple terms in a way that could be publicised to a general audience [up to 4000 chars]

There is a need to communicate and democratise recent innovation in UK engineering, and with this an opportunity to challenge and invigorate the public's perception of engineering. Unconventional collaboration methods used in PPE projects like Biojewellery and Robert Doubleday's sociological perspective on nanotechnology research are extended in this proposal, and employed to frame a creative and innovative process for representing the technical and sociocultural issues which attend engineering research, to a large and diverse audience.

This proposal responds to an emerging culture of joining up scientific, policy, critical and communication disciplines, and aims to challenge received PPE models. What distinguishes this proposal from the strategy of policy-focused engagement is that it aims to form collaborative networks which bring to life the detail and fascination of engineering in the imaginative worlds of an audience of end users.

The aim of this proposal is to pair experienced research engineers and designers through a residency program, leading to a series of public exhibitions and engagement events. These events will open up a reflective and critical space around the role of future technology, where the engineers' research can be represented to the public in a stimulating way

The proposal seeks to exploit the potential of engineer/designer partnerships, but it also seeks to extend the way imaginative and challenging outputs can have a large impact. It is anticipated that these outputs will be resonant for a range of discourses, and as a result be appropriated and constructively presented across a range of channels including print and TV media, academic journals, conferences and professional events, online forums, etc. The proposal aims to build new bridges between academic specialism and public engagement by pushing emotive and accessible formats.

Beneficiaries

Describe who will benefit from the research [up to 4000 chars].

There are three groupings of beneficiary, each group is a different scale and relationship with the outcomes:

Event audiences

Exhibition and event audiences, where the project outcomes are presented through exhibitions with larger museums (for example the V&A), and debates and encounters within the Dana Centre and Science Cafe's. The experience is structured around designed objects, writing, and documentation using film and photography. Other beneficiaries here include audiences reached as a result of unplanned participation in conferences as a result of invitation.

These beneficiaries are fairly quantifiable audiences linked to the visitor demographic of the participating venue or event Within the audiences of larger events like the V&A, particular groupings can be strategically targeted by tailoring the programming, by focussing on schools visits for example.

Media audiences

Other outcomes address audiences which are less defined and much larger, the aim is to provide broad coverage of the project at a national level. These beneficiaries are reached through press radio and TV media, papers and journals written by outside professionals, reviews and online chat. The project seeks to cultivate these outcomes throughout the project.

Participants

The third audience are the participants, and their peer groups. Along with the core engineers and designers and others working in the department where the collaborations are based, this includes members of the public invited to attend the reflection meetings, those participating in the design activity (as a test user for example) and other professionals and consultants attending and contributing to project events. This participant network has a direct influence on the development and outcome of the project, and will be those whose practices and experiences are most effected by engagement with the project.

Fig. I.3.2 *Material Beliefs proposal to EPSRC (page 2)*

1.4

MATERIAL BELIEFS IDENTITY BY HYPERKIT

The project had begun, but how to get going? We needed communication tools in order to initiate networks and invite collaboration. Hyperkit, a graphic design studio, created a typeface and logo, a website, stationery and templates for letters and posters – all arrived at this point, and enabled the project to move forward.

'Public engagement isn't something that we naturally wake up in the morning thinking about. So we do need someone to come in and say, "Why don't you try this or that type of activity?"'

TONY CASS
Institute of Biomedical Engineering, Imperial College London

'We created a hybrid typeface, to reflect the juxtapositions in the project: engineers/designers, machines/humans. We did this by cutting up two contrasting typefaces up and splicing the letters together.'

PETE SAMPSON
Graphic Designer, Hyperkit

Material
Beliefs

Fig. 1.4.1

abcdefghijklmnopqrstuvwxyz
ABCDEFGHIJKLMNOPQRSTUVWXYZ
0123456789

Fig. 1.4.2

1.4.1 *Material Beliefs logo*
1.4.2 *Typeface*

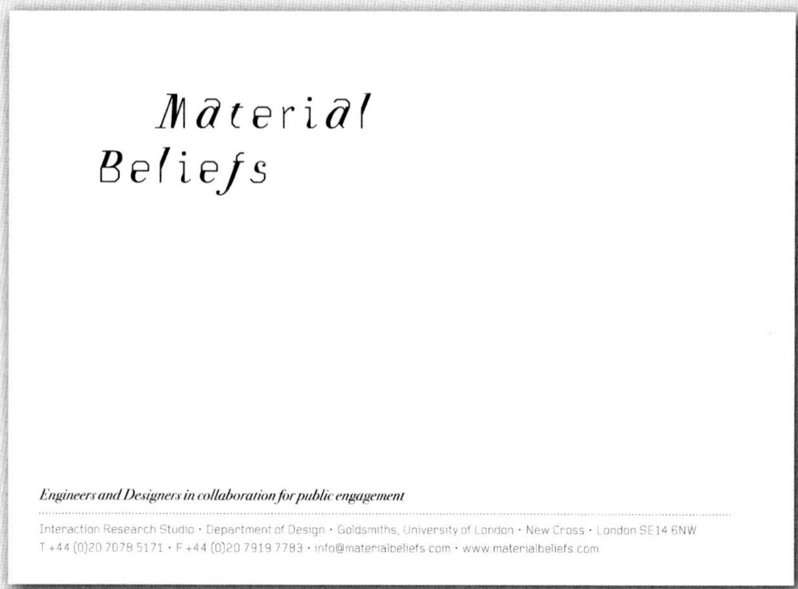

Material Beliefs

Engineers and Designers in collaboration for public engagement

Interaction Research Studio · Department of Design · Goldsmiths, University of London · New Cross · London SE14 6NW
T +44 (0)20 7078 5171 · F +44 (0)20 7919 7783 · info@materialbeliefs.com · www.materialbeliefs.com

Fig. 1.4.3

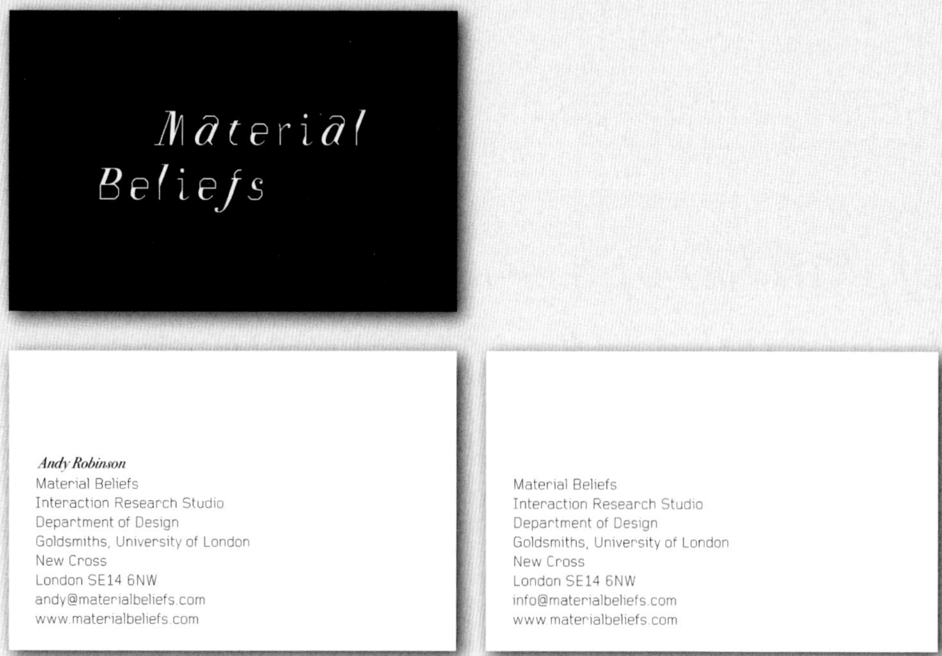

Andy Robinson
Material Beliefs
Interaction Research Studio
Department of Design
Goldsmiths, University of London
New Cross
London SE14 6NW
andy@materialbeliefs.com
www.materialbeliefs.com

Material Beliefs
Interaction Research Studio
Department of Design
Goldsmiths, University of London
New Cross
London SE14 6NW
info@materialbeliefs.com
www.materialbeliefs.com

Fig. 1.4.4

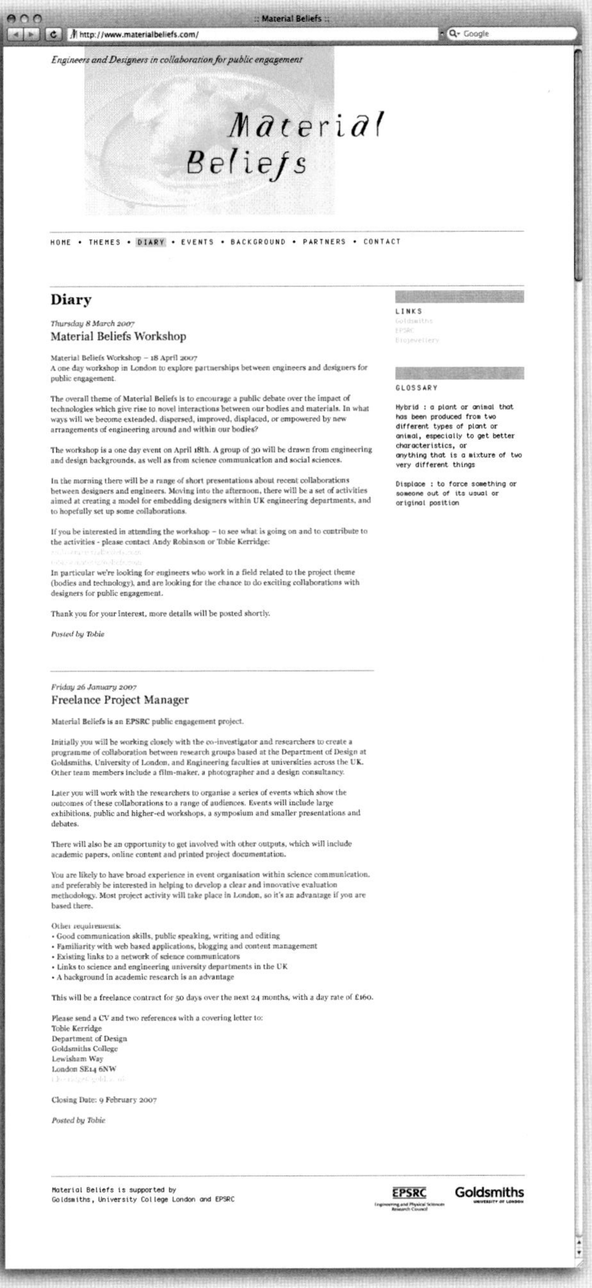

:: Material Beliefs ::

http://www.materialbeliefs.com/

Google

Engineers and Designers in collaboration for public engagement

Material Beliefs

HOME • THEMES • DIARY • EVENTS • BACKGROUND • PARTNERS • CONTACT

Diary

Thursday 8 March 2007

Material Beliefs Workshop

Material Beliefs Workshop – 18 April 2007
A one day workshop in London to explore partnerships between engineers and designers for public engagement.

The overall theme of Material Beliefs is to encourage a public debate over the impact of technologies which give rise to novel interactions between our bodies and materials. In what ways will we become extended, dispersed, improved, displaced, or empowered by new arrangements of engineering around and within our bodies?

The workshop is a one day event on April 18th. A group of 30 will be drawn from engineering and design backgrounds, as well as from science communication and social sciences.

In the morning there will be a range of short presentations about recent collaborations between designers and engineers. Moving into the afternoon, there will be a set of activities aimed at creating a model for embedding designers within UK engineering departments, and to hopefully set up some collaborations.

If you be interested in attending the workshop – to see what is going on and to contribute to the activities - please contact Andy Robinson or Tobie Kerridge:

In particular we're looking for engineers who work in a field related to the project theme (bodies and technology), and are looking for the chance to do exciting collaborations with designers for public engagement.

Thank you for your interest, more details will be posted shortly.

Posted by Tobie

Friday 26 January 2007

Freelance Project Manager

Material Beliefs is an EPSRC public engagement project.

Initially you will be working closely with the co-investigator and researchers to create a programme of collaboration between research groups based at the Department of Design at Goldsmiths, University of London, and Engineering faculties at universities across the UK. Other team members include a film-maker, a photographer and a design consultancy.

Later you will work with the researchers to organise a series of events which show the outcomes of these collaborations to a range of audiences. Events will include large exhibitions, public and higher-ed workshops, a symposium and smaller presentations and debates.

There will also be an opportunity to get involved with other outputs, which will include academic papers, online content and printed project documentation.

You are likely to have broad experience in event organisation within science communication, and preferably be interested in helping to develop a clear and innovative evaluation methodology. Most project activity will take place in London, so it's an advantage if you are based there.

Other requirements:
• Good communication skills, public speaking, writing and editing
• Familiarity with web based applications, blogging and content management
• Existing links to a network of science communicators
• Links to science and engineering university departments in the UK
• A background in academic research is an advantage

This will be a freelance contract for 50 days over the next 24 months, with a day rate of £160.

Please send a CV and two references with a covering letter to:
Tobie Kerridge
Department of Design
Goldsmiths College
Lewisham Way
London SE14 6NW

Closing Date: 9 February 2007

Posted by Tobie

LINKS
Goldsmiths
EPSRC
Biojewellery

GLOSSARY

Hybrid : a plant or animal that has been produced from two different types of plant or animal, especially to get better characteristics, or anything that is a mixture of two very different things

Displace : to force something or someone out of its usual or original position

Material Beliefs is supported by
Goldsmiths, University College London and EPSRC

EPSRC Engineering and Physical Sciences Research Council

Goldsmiths UNIVERSITY OF LONDON

Fig. 1.4.5

1.4.3 *Mailing label*
1.4.4 *Business cards*
1.4.5 *Website design*

1.5

COLLABORATION

WORKSHOP

The Collaboration Workshop, on 18 April 2007, was a one-day event held to explore partnerships between engineers and designers for public engagement. The 30 participants had backgrounds in engineering, science, design, social science and science communication. The next two pages show posters used at the workshop (featuring comments from invitees about their expectations for the day), and images and comments from the event.

Q: What do you consider to be the aims of Material Beliefs?

A: To discover connections and alliances, as well as friction points and paths of possibilities.

From the feedback form of a participant in the Collaboration Workshop

'The theme of play then became the key for us, and we started to talk about it as a methodology for creative practice. That led us to think about who we might work with, and how we might work with them, and we said that it was important to have time and space to allow things to grow.'

KAREN CHAM
During a feedback session at the Collaboration Workshop

Interesting things occur at the edges of fields of expertise

Material Beliefs pairs experienced research engineers and designers through a residency program. The aim of these reflective collaborations is to generate a body of work for public exhibition and engagement events. These events will open up a reflective and critical space around the role of future technology, in which the engineers' research can be represented to the public in a novel ways.

Wednesday 18 April 10am
The Women's Library
London Metropolitan University
Old Castle Street
London E1 7NT

info@materialbeliefs.com
www.materialbeliefs.com

Material Beliefs

EPSRC
Engineering and Physical Sciences
Research Council

Goldsmiths
UNIVERSITY OF LONDON

Fig. 1.5.1 *Collaboration Workshop poster*

THE
WORKSHOP

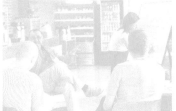

Fig. 1.5.2

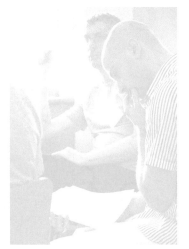

Fig. 1.5.3

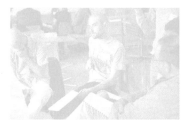

Fig. 1.5.4　　　　　　　　　　　　　　　　Fig. 1.5.5

Fig. 1.5.6

1.5.3 – 1.5.5 Workshop participants
1.5.6 Workshop materials

'At what stage do you want to engage the public? Do you want to bring people in throughout the entire collaboration, and not just wait until you get to the product at the end, and then do an exhibition?'
LESLEY PATERSON
During a feedback session at the Collaboration Workshop

'We started to talk about how you might set up this sort of collaboration, and who is served by what aspect of the collaboration. This means establishing a very clear idea of what outputs you wanted, how you were going to work, which part of the project served who, and what everybody might mean by publics and dissemination, and products or outputs.'
EMILY DAWSON
During a feedback session at the Collaboration Workshop

MATERIAL BELIEFS
INTERACTION RESEARCH STUDIO

1.6

INTERVIEWING RESEARCHERS

After the workshop, the collaboration leaders interviewed engineers and scientists in their labs. These were informal interviews, to find out in some detail about their work and interests, and identify points of crossover that could lead to collaboration. Four of the interviews had a big influence on the later design outcomes of Material Beliefs, and so are documented in the following pages. This chapter then ends with an extract from a guide to collaboration, written in order to clarify the expectations of potential participants in the project.

JIMMY: We went to Bristol initially, we went to Southampton, we went to all these places and they were very kind to show us their stuff and it was really invigorating, and what should have happened on that very same day is we should have –
JAMES: Given the design talk.
JIMMY: That would have saved months of rejection issues [laughs].

JIMMY LOIZEAU   AND   JAMES AUGER
Department of Design, Goldsmiths   *Design Interactions, Royal College of Art*

'I acknowledge that the way one works in an entirely different discipline may almost require the absence of planning to achieve an objective. However, you can't have the design side, if that is less driven by deadline and planning, assuming that the science can just follow along in some similar way, because it just ain't going to happen. You can't throw things into an open schedule and see what grows. That was my concern.'

BEN WHALLEY
The University of Reading, School of Pharmacy

1.6.1 *Kevin Warwick interviewed at the University of Reading*

Kevin Warwick is Professor of Cybernetics at the University of Reading, where he carries out research in artificial intelligence, control, robotics and biomedical engineering.

As a part of the Cybernetics Group, Warwick has carried out a series of pioneering experiments involving the neurosurgical implantation of a device into the median nerves of his left arm. This provided a link between his nervous system and a computer, offering a prototype system for a range of potential applications.

He has been successful with the first extra-sensory (ultrasonic) input for a human, and with the first purely electronic communication experiment between the nervous systems of two humans. He is currently working on a new project involving the implementation of neural tissue, to provide a feedback loop from the tissue to a small robot called Miobot.

His research has been widely discussed by the news media coverage and special interest groups, and featured in the White House Presidential Council on Bioethics.

KEVIN WARWICK

Fig. 1.6.1

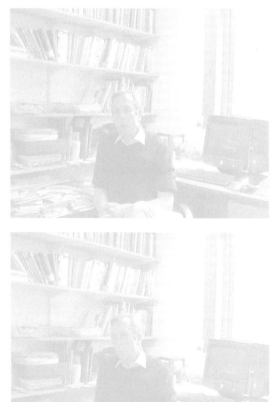

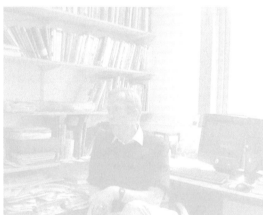

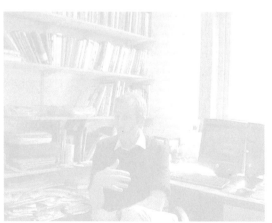

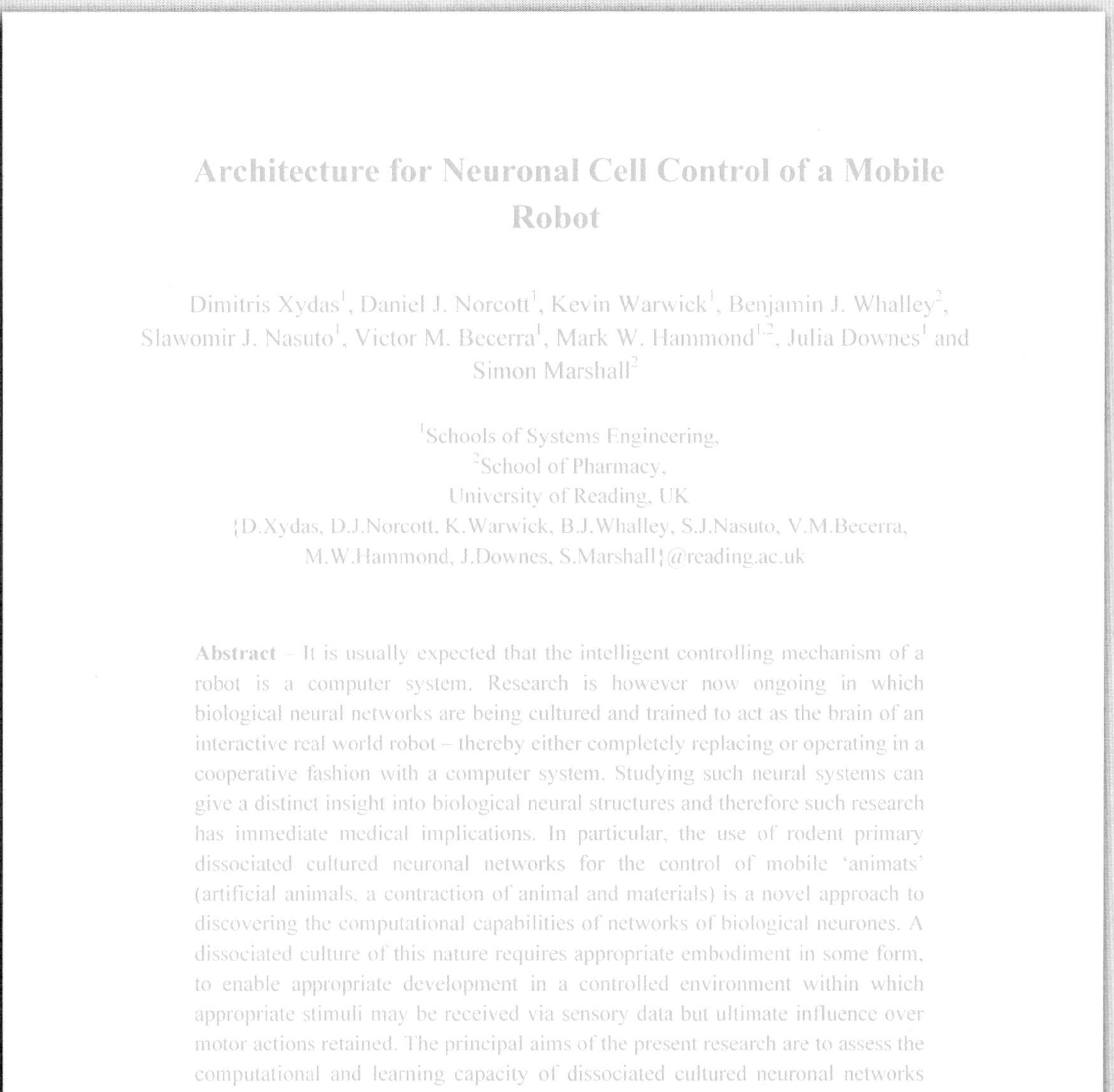

Architecture for Neuronal Cell Control of a Mobile Robot

Dimitris Xydas[1], Daniel J. Norcott[1], Kevin Warwick[1], Benjamin J. Whalley[2], Slawomir J. Nasuto[1], Victor M. Becerra[1], Mark W. Hammond[1,2], Julia Downes[1] and Simon Marshall[2]

[1]Schools of Systems Engineering,
[2]School of Pharmacy,
University of Reading, UK
{D.Xydas, D.J.Norcott, K.Warwick, B.J.Whalley, S.J.Nasuto, V.M.Becerra, M.W.Hammond, J.Downes, S.Marshall}@reading.ac.uk

Abstract – It is usually expected that the intelligent controlling mechanism of a robot is a computer system. Research is however now ongoing in which biological neural networks are being cultured and trained to act as the brain of an interactive real world robot – thereby either completely replacing or operating in a cooperative fashion with a computer system. Studying such neural systems can give a distinct insight into biological neural structures and therefore such research has immediate medical implications. In particular, the use of rodent primary dissociated cultured neuronal networks for the control of mobile 'animats' (artificial animals, a contraction of animal and materials) is a novel approach to discovering the computational capabilities of networks of biological neurones. A dissociated culture of this nature requires appropriate embodiment in some form, to enable appropriate development in a controlled environment within which appropriate stimuli may be received via sensory data but ultimate influence over motor actions retained. The principal aims of the present research are to assess the computational and learning capacity of dissociated cultured neuronal networks with a view to advancing network level processing of artificial neural networks. This will be approached by the creation of an artificial hybrid system (animat) involving closed loop control of a mobile robot by a dissociated culture of rat neurons. This 'closed loop' interaction with the environment through both sensing and effecting will enable investigation of its learning capacity This paper details the components of the overall animat closed loop system and reports on the evaluation of the results from the experiments being carried out with regard to robot behaviour.

Key words: Dissociated neurones, robotic animats, culture stimulation, neural plasticity

Fig. 1.6.2 *Academic paper describing neuronal control of a robot*

Fig. 1.6.3

TRACKING AND MONITORING

KEVIN

About five years ago we looked into the possibility of using implant technology for tracking and monitoring people. It was the time of the Soham murders, and at that time there was a considerable ethical backlash against technology for tracking children ... using technology, worn, maybe as a watch or like a tag, or an implant, for locating somebody, within a matter of seconds to within a few metres.

A local newsagency came up and said we have this 11-year-old girl and her parents and they are happy to let her [be tracked]. But what happened is a backlash. The NSPCC in the UK said it was a terrible thing. Children's societies came out very negatively. Abduction was pushed to one side and technology was the negative thing. So I backed out.

It's very difficult to know, as a technical person, what to do – so I answer them, yes, technically it is possible if people wanted this for their child, they could put an armband on. It will be interesting five or six years on from the Soham case how society has moved ethically. I'm not making any claims that yes, I'm going to do that with this child, but it will be interesting to see.

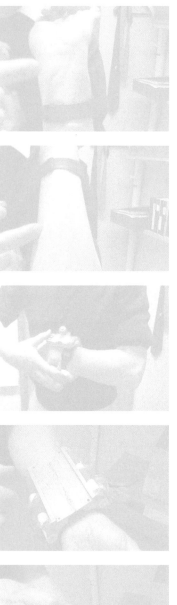

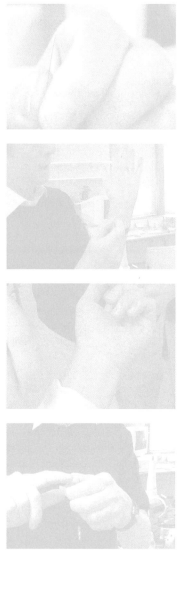

Fig. 1.6.4

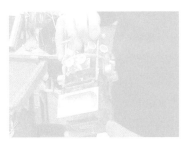
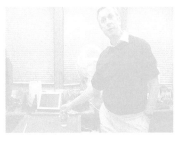

ROBOT BRAIN

KEVIN
This robot will be the first to have a biological brain.

Currently it has a brain of 30,000-50,000 neurons. What if, next year, it has a brain of 1,000,000,000 neurons? You are up to the level of a dog or a pretty intelligent cat. So should it have the rights of an animal? Do we need to have a licence to look after it? And how should we look after it?

If this has the same brain as a dog, OK, it doesn't look like a dog, it doesn't pee like a dog, it doesn't do things that dogs do - but maybe it will. Maybe with ten million neurons it will start becoming sexually attached to my right leg.

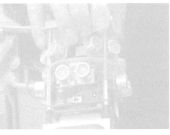
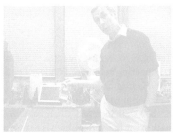
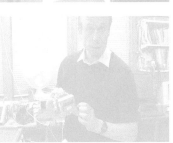
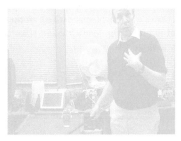
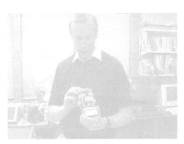
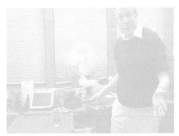

1.6.3 *Kevin Warwick describing how electrodes were inserted into his arm*
1.6.4 *Kevin Warwick with a Miobot*

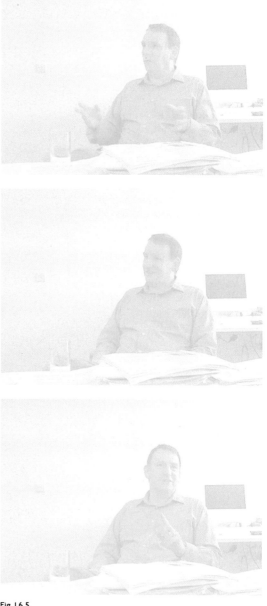

TONY CASS

Tony Cass is Deputy Director of the Institute of Biomedical Engineering at Imperial College London.

Having originally trained as a chemist, Cass is also a Professor of Chemical Biology at Imperial, and a Fellow of the Royal Society of Chemistry. We focused on his work within the institute, which is based in a new facility aimed at fostering a multidisciplinary research environment. It creates a physical space where workers from the faculties of Engineering, Medicine and Natural Sciences can meet and share resources.

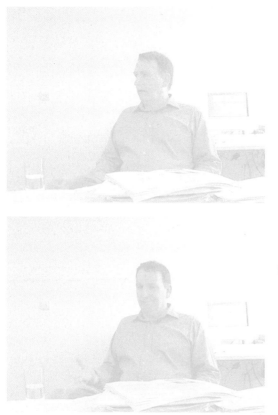

Fig. 1.6.5

1.6.5 *Tony Cass interviewed at the Institute of Biomedical Engineering*

Ultra-low power UWB for real time biomedical wireless sensing

Chun Yi Lee and Christofer Toumazou

Institute of Biomedical Engineering,

Imperial College London

ABSTRACT : ISFET, MEMS and advances in semiconductor technology have enabled the realization of powerful miniature devices for physiological signal monitoring. Sensors are becoming very small with amazingly low power consumption. They can measure a wide range of physiological signal, e.g. ECG, EEG, blood glucose level, blood oxygen level, etc. The integration of those devices, low power signal processing and ultra low power (ULP) wireless telemetry creates the synergy that has never been explored. Prolong real time physiological signal monitoring can be achieved more easily and economically. Conventional ULP wireless telemetry systems are approaching their lower bound on power consumption. Ultra Wideband (UWB) communication system can probably break the limit because of its simple architecture and carrier-free characteristic. The power consumption and chip size per unit of data rate can be made very low. More room for tradeoffs in the system is allowed.

I. INTRODUCTION

Aging population problem has been reported in developed countries and the situation is becoming worse. The cost of running a public health system is increasing in many countries. Remote patients monitoring system [1], [2] is believed to be a moderate solution to the problem by sending patients home and monitoring with a centrally connected management system. Body temperature, blood pressure, ECG and EEG are the information or signals with vital importance to doctors.

Usually, wires connect the sensor body to a processing or recording unit. Power is delivered to the sensor circuits through the wire and the acquired data is collected simultaneously. Though the use of wire solves two problems at one time, it becomes problematic for long term host monitoring.

Real time continuous physiological signal monitoring is necessary to capture abnormalities occasionally happen in our body. For example, heartthrob and heart beat rate irregularity, they are difficult to be identified as they last for a short period of time. Long term ECG monitoring has to be carried out in order to capture these irregularities. Usually, the patient is asked to wear a set of wired surface electrodes with a recording device in his daily life for several days.

Acknowledge financial support of ETSRC grant number GR/R9658/01

The wires connecting the electrodes to the recording device usually cause signal integrity problem and inconvenience to the host. When the host moves, vibrations propagate along the wires and reach the electrodes. The skin-electrode contact impedance varies. Noise or known as artifacts may be resulted in the acquired signals. The situation will be even more severe if the host is required to do exercise during the test. The hosts cannot move freely with the wires, which adversely affect their daily life.

To exploit the true potential of a wireless real time physiological signal monitoring system on an off hospital patient monitoring system, the wire between the sensor body and the recording device must be removed. With the state-of-the-art semiconductor technology, MEMS and ISFET, etc, the size of a sensor is shrinking as well as its power consumption. High processing power is available with minimal amount of power consumption and a larger variety of physical parameters can be accessed directly by semiconductor devices. The only missing part is an ultra low power wireless telemetry link between the sensor body and the recording device. In this paper, we will investigate the possibility of replacing the wires with an Ultra Wideband communication system. The corresponding advantages will be discussed in detail.

II. SENSOR ARCHITECTURE

General sensor architecture can be depicted as Figure 1.

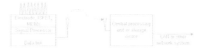

Figure 1 General architecture of a smart sensor system

The front end of the sensor is the interface of the semiconductor chip and the physical world. Microelectrodes, membrane of an ISFET and micromechanical structure are useful to collect the necessary information. The acquired signals are usually weak and contaminated with noise. Certain simple signal pre-processing has to be carried out to reject unwanted signal and condition the raw signal. In some special cases, pre-processing is preferable to be carried out at the site the signal is acquired. For example, an artificial retina[3] has a large number of signal inputs, automatic gain control and edge searching are carried out at the front end sensing elements. This is a good example of bio inspired electronic design.

Fig. 1.6.6 *Academic paper describing low power biometric sensors*

Fig. 1.6.7

Fig. 1.6.8

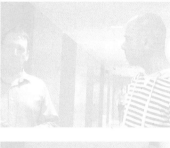

BIOMEDICAL ENGINEERING

TONY
Scale is important. We intervene on two scales. One is small scale, millimetres, essentially surgery – cutting, slicing, and stitching. Then you've got the molecular scale: pharmaceuticals. In between those two – cells, tissues – is less developed. Between the scalpel and the pill – that's where a lot of the interesting new developments in the scale of things are coming about.

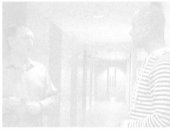

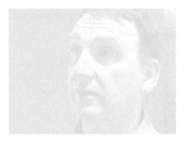

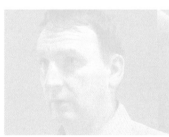

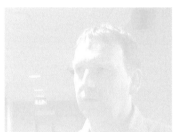

SETTING UP THE INSTITUTE OF BIOMEDICAL ENGINEERING

TONY
What we wanted was to create some space that would make it easy for people to move in, to work together, and then to move back to their own department. And space where you could mix up electrical engineers, cardiologists, molecular biologists...

Researchers have to be engaged in the areas that we have identified as interesting in biomedical engineering, so that's things like tissue engineering, medical robotics, bionics (which is the use of silicon electronics in biomedical devices), and nanotechnology and its applications to healthcare. We try and be as open as possible to people coming in.

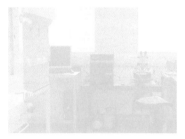

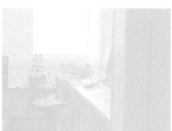

1.6.7 *Tony Cass and Elio Caccavale*
1.6.8 *Institute of Biomedical Engineering*
1.6.9 *Nanofabrication facility*
1.6.10 *Da Vinci robotic medical assistant*

MATERIAL BELIEFS
INTERACTION RESEARCH STUDIO

Fig. 1.6.9

Fig. 1.6.10

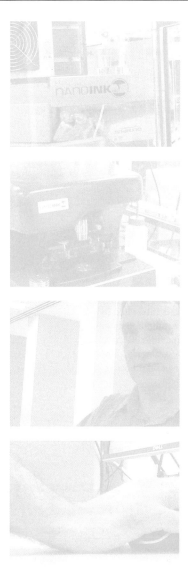

ENGINEERING AND SCIENCE

TONY

Engineers are scientists who like to build things. If you think traditional science is describing how the world works, understanding how the world works, engineering is understanding how the world works and then using that understanding to change the world. So if you like, the physics of gravity is understanding how gravity works, but the engineering of aeronautics is understanding how gravity works and then building machines that overcome gravity, that mean you can fly.

That's what we're best at doing, taking quantitative data and then interpreting it – not necessarily saying to someone 'your blood pressure (on the monitor) is 150 over 30', or whatever, but saying 'your blood pressure is too high'. There is a whole area of presenting hard quantitative data to the public – how you translate numerical data and present it to people.

NANOTECH

TONY

The nanotech community is very conscious of not belittling public concern, because what one wants to do is explain the advantages, acknowledge the potential hazards – and these are in many cases unknown materials, so they are potential hazards...

The thing you always hear is 'we don't want to go down the GM crops route', which in many ways was a perfectly safe technology with many benefits, but the people who were primarily promoting it rejected the public concerns, which was a complete disaster. So even if on a technical scientific level the concerns are unfounded, they have to be treated with respect.

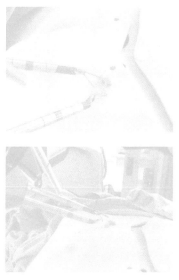

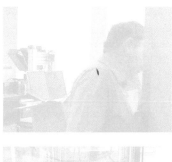

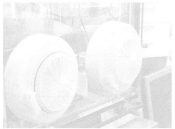

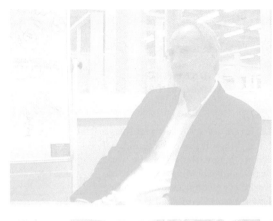

CHRIS MELHUISH

Bristol Robotics Laboratory is based at a new facility in Bristol Business Park. The lab focusses on bioengineering and intelligent autonomous systems, and aims to understand the science, engineering and social role of robotics and embedded intelligence.

Chris Melhuish is the director at BRL, which has over 50 members of staff and students. He is interested in making robot systems which can behave autonomously in an intelligent manner. His research areas include collective as well as single robot systems, energy autonomy, biologically based neuro-controllers and humanoid robots.

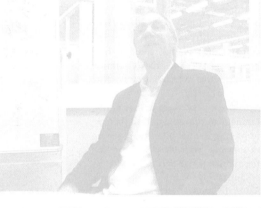

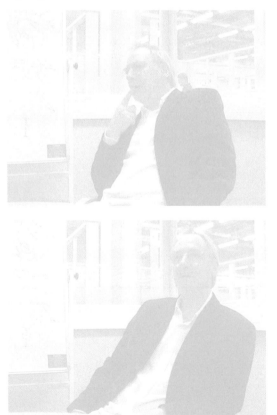

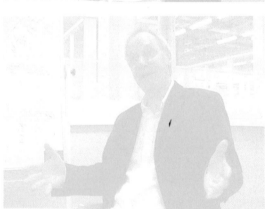

Fig. 1.6.11

1.6.11 *Chris Melhuish interviewed at Bristol Robotics Lab*

In Proceedings of the AISB '03, Second
International Symposium on Imitation
in Animals and Artifacts,
Aberystwyth, Wales, pp 191-4, 2003.

Imitating Metabolism: Energy Autonomy in Biologically Inspired Robots

Ioannis Ieropoulos[1]   John Greenman[2]   Chris Melhuish[1]

[1]IAS Lab, CEMS Faculty   [2]Faculty of Applied Sciences   [1]IAS Lab, CEMS Faculty
UWE, Coldharbour Lane, Frenchay, Bristol, UWE, Coldharbour Lane, Frenchay, Bristol, UWE, Coldharbour Lane, Frenchay, Bristol,
BS16 1QY, UK   BS16 1QY, UK   BS16 1QY, UK
Ioannis2.Ieropoulos@uwe.ac.u   John.Greenman@uwe.ac.uk   Chris.Melhuish@uwe.ac.uk

Abstract

This paper reports on the initial work to produce an artificial metabolic system for an energetically autonomous robot using a Microbial Fuel Cell (MFC). We describe the fuel cell developed in our laboratory and demonstrate that it is feasible to provide sufficient power for a mobile robot platform to execute photo tactic 'pulsed' behaviour.

1 Introduction

The term 'autonomous robot' has been ascribed to robotic systems to indicate their ability to perform tasks without human supervision. In fact, from the ancient times, people have attempted to build machines, which could operate without direct control. For example, in 60 A.D. Heron of Alexandria built, possibly, the first recorded example of an automaton [1]. This was a self-moving cart, driven by a counter-weight that was attached to the wheeled base axles through ropes. However, the term 'autonomous' is somewhat flexible in that it covers degrees of autonomy. For example, consider the case of a robot whose batteries are charged by a human and then released to carry out its task without further external intervention. On completion of the task or in the event of the battery charge becoming critically low the robot returns to a base for recharging and/or new instructions. On one hand certain aspects of the robot's behaviour may be considered as autonomous; computational and control decisions are made without human supervision. On the other hand, without a human in the loop, the robot would not be able to replenish its energy to accomplish the task. With this in mind our long-term goal is the creation of a robot, which can generate energy for itself from its own environment. That energy could, for example, come from solar energy or even wind energy. Our interest however, is in generating energy from chemical substrate – food. We are therefore interested in a class of robot system, which demonstrates energetic autonomy by converting natural raw chemical substrate (such as carrots or apples) into power for essential elements of behaviour including motion, sensing and computation. This requires an artificial digestion system and concomitant artificial metabolism.

Adopting such a strategy may have an impact on the manner in which researchers and engineers incorporate their autonomous mission requirements. Three key issues are; firstly, useful energy will not (for the foreseeable future) be able to be instantly converted from raw substrate and secondly, there will be tasks (particularly those involving effectors or motion) which could not be powered continuously. The net effect is that this class of robot may have to include a 'waiting' behaviour in its repertoire in order to accumulate sufficient energy to carry out a task or sub-task. We refer to this form of behaviour as 'pulsed behaviour'. Thirdly, a robot may need to solve multi-goal action selection problems. In particular, it may be required to exhibit 'opportunistic' behaviour in terms of breaking off from its mission to forage or take advantage of energy resources such as a fallen apple. In nature, animals, in the wild, often exhibit such behaviours and our work is obviously biologically inspired at the metabolic and behavioural levels.

2 Microbial Fuel Cell

The idea of employing microbes to extract energy from sugars has been known for many years [2]. Raw substrate can be converted to sugars and then used in a Microbial Fuel Cell (MFC); a *bio-*electrochemical transducer that converts *bio-*chemical energy to electrical energy. The MFC, shown in Figure 1, comprises anode and cathode

Fig. 1.6.12 *Academic paper describing the use of microbial fuel cells in robots*

Fig. 1.6.13

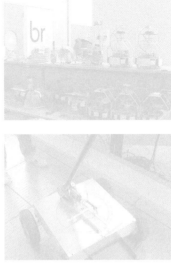

RESEARCH PORTFOLIO

CHRIS
The portfolio of the lab is fairly broad. We include work from collective robotics to human-robot interaction. For example, we worked with neuroscientists to produce analogues of neural architectures on silicon. We're interested in machines that can be self-sustaining and we're also engaged with autonomous systems that can go under water and in the air too. We have a fairly hefty programme of public engagement of science as well.

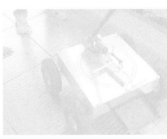

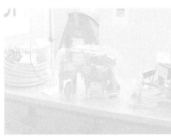

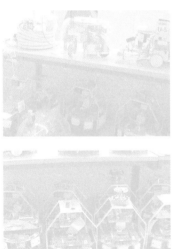

Fig. 1.6.14

HUBRIS AND CONNOTATIONS

CHRIS
Although we have confederations of British Industry, we have to be looking at where we are going to be in 30 years time. I still see, from time to time, this post-colonial hubris: we are all so creative in this country, you know. But what do we actually make? I'm being extreme here to make the point. But in truth the creative bit and the making bit are not really separate. They need to be joined together because there are iterative loops that you need to go round – you need to understand the materials that you're being creative with. Let's not kid ourselves that we have some sort of special creative gift

in the UK, because we don't. That's something that I think we should be cautioned against – hubris.

Engineering is still lumbered with being boring, with being male, still seen as being Victorian, or post-Victorian – men wearing white coats with spanners and slide-rules. That's not what modern engineering is, certainly in our area. It's far more creative and involved with science, as in trying to discover either how systems work, or how new materials can improve. There are a lot of questions we can ask, not simply, 'What do you want? We can make it for you'. So engineering has got to work hard at changing that image.

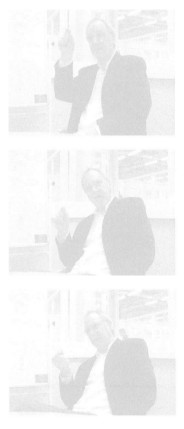

1.6.13 *Bristol Robotics Lab*
1.6.14 *Chris Melhuish interviewed at Bristol Robotics Lab*

CHRIS MASON

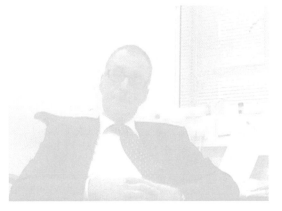

Professor Chris Mason is at the forefront of the emerging field of stem cell and regenerative medicine translation and commercialisation.

Chris has a background in basic science, clinical medicine, bioprocessing and business. He holds a Clinical Sciences degree, a degree in Medicine, and a PhD in tissue-engineering bioprocessing from University College London, where he currently works.

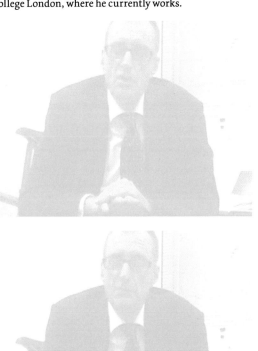

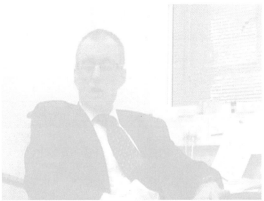

Fig. 1.6.15

1.6.15 *Chris Mason interviewed at University College London*

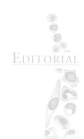

A brief definition of regenerative medicine

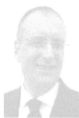

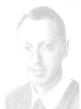

*Chris Mason[1] &
Peter Dunnill*

*[1]Author for correspondence
Advanced Centre for
Biochemical Engineering,
University College London,
London WC1E 7JE, UK
Tel.: +44 207 679 0140;
Fax: +44 207 209 0703;
E-mail: chris.mason@
ucl.ac.uk*

'There are already a lot of definitions, but all are lengthy and not the sort of thing scientists, start-ups or advocates can say succinctly when a pharma executive, government minister or member of the public asks for clarification.'

While it could be said that regenerative medicine is what this journal publishes, that would be cyclical. It could also be claimed that most people interested in the field have a good grasp of what is entailed, and this is probably correct. But, as the field grows and there is a need to carry governments and public opinion along, it is probably worth having a simple explanation of regenerative medicine. And, it is simplicity that is the nub of the matter. There are already a lot of definitions [1–3] but all are lengthy and not the sort of thing scientists, start-ups or advocates can say succinctly when a pharma executive, government minister or member of the public asks for clarification. Here, we address this and the origins and relationships that help to define the field.

One of the complications is that regenerative medicine has grown out of a good deal of prior activity. This includes surgery, surgical implants, such as artificial hips, and increasingly sophisticated biomaterial scaffolds. It also draws on hospital procedures such as bone marrow and organ transplants and it relates to tissue engineering. There is no absolute cut-off in the transformation of these into fully developed regenerative medicine but they each leave residues of their input that can mean the patient is not capable of being termed 'of natural health' with respect to the treated condition. Organ transplants often demand immune-suppressing drugs and metal hips can become loose with time, engineered tissue scaffolds can provoke inflammation and bone marrow sources are variable mixtures that also can be contaminated quite easily by the nature of the cell aspiration procedure.

The central focus of regenerative medicine is human cells. These may be somatic, adult stem or embryo-derived cells and now there are versions of the latter cells that have been reprogrammed from adult cells so that both can be conveniently collected under the heading of 'pluripotent cells' [4,5]. There appears to be a progression in interest through this sequence. It is driven by the limitations in availability of most specialist somatic cells and the restriction in the expansion of adult stem cells together with their heterogeneity from sources such as bone marrow. Human embryos are not an ideal source from a technical point of view, leaving aside the ethical and moral issues. For this reason, obtaining pluripotent cells in another way is attractive. This progression entails the transfer of genes to human cells [6] and this could bring regenerative medicine and gene therapy closer.

Though inevitably the pioneering phase leading towards regenerative medicine has been marked by some failures, there are now sound commercial products for skin ulcer and sports injury damage to the cartilage of the knee [7]. There are also exciting developments with respect to treating patients with bladder dysfunction [8]. These therapies use either autologous or allogeneic somatic cells and, in the case of skin and bladder, the products have a biomaterials component. The outcome of therapy with adult stem cells is at present less clear because the status of these cells is being debated [9], but in the end it will be proof or otherwise of therapeutic outcome that defines their importance.

'In the medium term, there are a number of major medical conditions, such as heart failure, insulin-dependant diabetes, spinal cord injury, Parkinson's and possibly Alzheimer's diseases, which appear to be addressable via cell-based therapies.'

For the present, most of the developments with embryo-derived cells are as pure cell therapies, although treatment of age-related macular degeneration is likely to involve a scaffold [10]. It is probable that in time more therapies involving embryonic stem cells and temporary scaffolds will appear and certainly where structural tissue is demanded it is hard to see cells

10.2217/17460751.3.1.1 © 2008 Future Medicine Ltd ISSN 1746-0751

Fig. 1.6.16 *Editorial overview of regenerative medicine*

Fig. 1.6.17

REGENERATIVE MEDICINE

CHRIS
In my lab we're looking at toxicology, really, with the stem cell sciences project. We're asking if you can grow human cells at quantity, using robotics to produce high numbers. Pharmaceutical companies are interested in it, but it's still five to ten years away from being routine ...

We are very close to therapies for spinal cord injuries, for certain types of blindness. It would be crazy to discontinue those programmes now when we are so close to delivering real benefits to patients with those therapies.

In the future, ten years from now, we will no longer be using embryonic stem cell lines. We will be using cells taken from the skin and reprogrammed. This is politically and ethically more acceptable, and probably easier to use. If we wanted to make a specific disease model, for example – let's say I've got early on-set Huntington's disease. Then take a few cells from me and you've got the model for early on-set Huntington's disease. You know I've got it, whereas when we take these embryonic stem cell lines ...well, we've no idea.

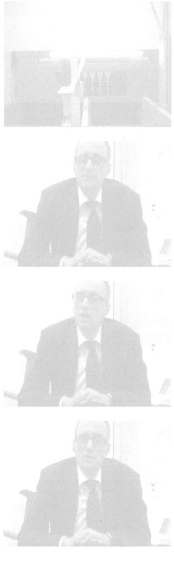

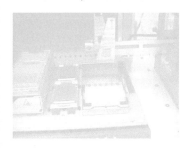

Fig. 1.6.18

PERSONALISED MEDICINE

CHRIS
It comes down to this thing called 'personalised medicine'. We're not going to see big blockbuster drugs in the future because the data has shown us that probably the drugs only work in a half to two-thirds of the patients anyway, and in another half to two-thirds they have side effects. What you really want to do, in the dream scenario – you go along to your doctor, and he says, 'this is what is wrong with you', he says, 'this is a great drug', and then tests it on a chip with appropriate human cells to see if the drug would have any effect on you, and he would also check it on a liver cell chip to ensure it was safe. So he'd test for efficacy and safety, and only when he's done that could he prescribe the drug for you.

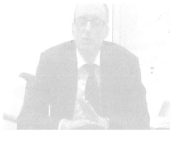

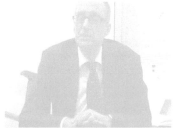

1.6.17 *An automated laboratory liquid handling system*
1.6.18 *Chris Mason interviewed at University College London*

Material Beliefs Collaborations

This document is designed to provide a guide for setting-up collaborations between designers and engineering groups.

Material Beliefs aims to:
– Enable scientists and engineers to build links between their research activity and cultural institutions.
– Challenge the working methods of designers by deepening their experience of science and engineering.
– Embed engineering research within material culture, so that a broad audience can interpret it.
– Develop innovative models of engagement between science and the everyday, academia and the publics.

Benefits

There are a range of benefits and opportunities for these collaborations. It's important that there are clear benefits for everyone involved, and these should be discussed at the outset. For the department/research group there is a chance to work collaboratively on a public engagement project with a group of outside professionals. This will put the research in front of a range of potentially new audiences, and to a broad network of other academics and professionals. For individuals there is a chance to stand back from the focus of their research, and see their work differently, and how it is interpreted by others. The collaboration is likely to offer support for engagement activities they have wanted to do but not started. There will also be opportunities to promote work with others.

Time-scale

The collaboration takes place over a one year period, leading to a series of exhibition and public engagement events in autumn 2008. The funding period ends in December 2008. It is imagined that there are two broad phases to the collaboration: the first half is exploratory and the second half is about making.

Resources

Material Beliefs has a financial package of up to £5000 for each collaborating department. This can be used by the collaborating group to help meet costs. This might include buying out some of the researchers time and travel, contributing towards consumable costs or equipment hire.

Work-plan

A plan of work should be negotiated between collaborators. This will be discussed at the outset, and though it is likely to change, it helps manage expectations. It's also worth thinking about who will be the main point of contact, and who else within the department will be a part of the collaboration, including researchers, technicians and students. The collaboration might fall anywhere within a range of contact and involvement, from occasional visits and meetings, to residencies.

Outcomes, Accuracy and Copyright

The project would work towards a range of outcomes, including designed objects, writing, and documentation using film and photography, to be presented at exhibitions, via the project website, at higher education seminars and workshops, and at larger live discussion events. It's also important to have a clear picture of how the work is being disseminated, and that everyone is happy about these outputs. This might be negotiated as opportunities arise, and continue beyond the projects timeframe.

Evaluation

The evaluation process will complement the collaborative nature of the project. Collaborators will use the project website to record their processes of research and public engagement. It will provide both a space for internal evaluation and link them to exhibition and event partners, industry and members of the public. The Project Manager will structure a process with collaborators that creates agreed success criteria and indicators. It will focus on determining what questions need to be asked at each stage of the project to explore success, and what processes and outcomes are recorded and shared throughout the project.

Fig. 1.6.19 *Extract from a guide to setting up collaborations*

Chapter 2

A CARNIVOROUS FLY-EATING KETTLE

—

ENGAGING PEOPLE

2.0

A CARNIVOROUS
FLY-EATING KETTLE
–
ENGAGING
PEOPLE

'Being asked about the process rather than the product can be disorientating.'
TONY CASS
Institute of Biomedical Engineering, Imperial College London

'We've had great fun. We've had prototypes in two and three dimensions. We've had robots that use honey to trap flies, robots that use spiders to trap flies, and some generally quite nasty robots. Oh, and we've had a carnivorous fly-eating kettle.'
JIMMY LOIZEAU
Department of Design, Goldsmiths, at Family Fun Day, Royal Institute of Great Britain

The Café Scientifique movement was founded in Leeds in 1998, on the model of the French Café Philosophique, a grassroots forum for philosophical discussion which began in Paris in the early 1990s. There are now over 200 Café Scientifiques across the world, 30 of them in Britain. It was in places like the Café Scientifique in Newcastle, and the Science Museum's Dana Centre, that we first put designers and engineers on stage together. The idea was to take both parties out of their respective labs, away from the site of their embedded notions – to loosen up, have a beer, get talking. Could we begin to generate a shared language out of shared interests?

We discussed our work with the audiences, and fielded questions about the practicalities and ethics of silicon/cell hybrid technologies. How might humans, and other potentially hybrid life forms, behave in the future? In what ways might prosthetic body parts, wearable body extensions and smart textiles improve, empower, confine, displace or disperse us?

For the engineers, the challenge was to invite debate without pre-empting their research through overly bold or misleading claims. For the designers, questions about the future begged a more immediate question: how should we describe the relationship between the outcomes of research and our experiences of change?

This chapter ends with an account of Biotech, a short collaborative project which took engineers and design students far away from the public stage, to the mundane – or perhaps exotic? – private world of the lab.

2.1

EARLY PUBLIC
ENGAGEMENT
EVENTS

One way of transforming the energy of the collaborations into public engagement formats at this early stage was to partner with event organisers. The following documentation brings together photography, film stills and comment from four partnerships of this kind: a presentation to year nine students as part of the *Junior Scientifique* programme at the Thomas Hepburn Community School outside Newcastle; a discussion later that day as part of *Cyborg Debate: Our Future Human Body* at Newcastle's Cafe Scientifique; a summer workshop for young people, *My Space, My City, My World*, at the Stephen Lawrence Centre in South London; and a foray into the *Guerrilla Science Camp*, part of the Secret Garden Festival in the Cambridgeshire countryside.

'There's a culture in science to not shoot your mouth off, and to prove something several times in-house before you even think about taking it anywhere.'

NICK OLIVER
Institute of Biomedical Engineering, Imperial College London

'It seems to me that if you've got a potentially very powerful technology, a good way to make bad things happen is to restrict access to a small number of people.'

ADRIAN BOWER
Department of Mechanical Engineering, University of Bath

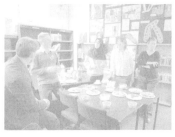

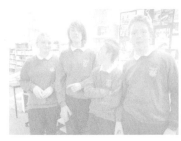

2.1.1 *Staff and students at the Thomas Hepburn Community School, with Patrick from Imperial College and Steve, a documentary film-maker*
2.1.2 *Students at the Thomas Hepburn Community School*
2.1.3 *Patrick discusses bionic vision systems*
2.1.4 *Tobie discusses tissue engineering*

Fig. 2.1.1

Fig. 2.1.2

JUNIOR SCIENTIFIQUE

—

THE THOMAS HEPBURN COMMUNITY SCHOOL

'Thank you from all concerned for yesterday's Café. Sorry there were not more kids there, but there's an issue with not being seen as 'swots' and not staying behind. The ones who were there thought it was great and have been talking about it today. There could be a market in a few years for bone jewellery!'
CLAIRE HARRISON
School Librarian, The Thomas Hepburn Community School

Fig. 2.1.3

Fig. 2.1.4

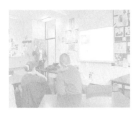
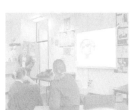
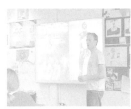
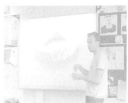

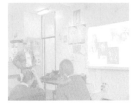
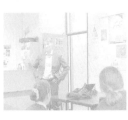
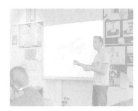
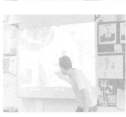

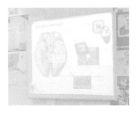
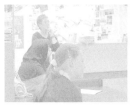
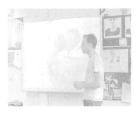
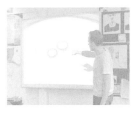

Evaluation Collation

Gender   Male   [3]   Female   [4]

Year Group   7   [ ]   8   [ ]   9   [6]   10   [ ]   11   [1]

What did you think about this session?

Excellent [6]   Good [1]   Ok [ ]   Poor [ ]   Very Poor [ ]

What did you think of the speaker?   (tick as many boxes as you like)

Interesting [6]   Funny [4]   Boring [ ]   Too old [ ]   Too young [ ]

Talked too much [1]   Didn't talk enough [ ]

Other

Which part did you like best?

Food and Drinks [ ]   Group discussions [2]   Listening to the speaker [5]

Arguing for your views [ ]   Listening to other people's ideas [2]

Will you attend the next meeting?

Yes [7]   No [ ]   Not sure [ ]

What do you think needs to be improved?

Need it to be longer.

Fig. 2.1.5 *Junior Scientifique feedback form*

Fig. 2.1.6

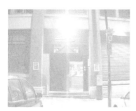

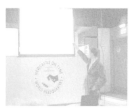

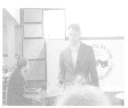

PATRICK DEGENAAR
Imperial College London
Are bionic eyes possible? We believe so. In my research group, we aim to stimulate the remaining neural tissue of degenerate eyes with light rather than electricity. Because that will cost a lot less power, we'd possibly be able to develop our approach into something small and compact like a pair of glasses.

TOBIE KERRIDGE
Goldsmiths
When we think of cyborg bodies we often think of ourselves as being augmented, or extended, or fixed. But, of course, we can also think of biological systems being put into everyday objects. This for me is something interesting, not just for the potential applications, but because, as a designer, I might be able to use the idea to provoke debate on the social value of this technology.

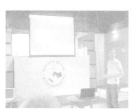

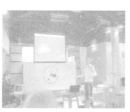

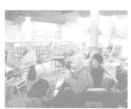

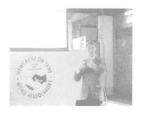

2.1.6 *Film stills from Cyborgs at Newcastle Café Scientifique*

CYBORG DEBATE
—
CAFÉ SCIENTIFIQUE

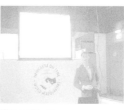

DISCUSSANT
Café Scientifique
To me, this seems like a crucial question: whether in using these technologies you're bringing a deficit up to normal performance or whether you are using technology to enhance beyond normal performance? There was a time when the NHS produced only one kind of spectacle for people; now of course you can wear lenses, flexible lenses, breathable lenses, disposable lenses, you could possibly have surgery to correct the lens in your eye. Is it the case that when we are looking for a stick or a crutch for a serious impairment, we'll tolerate poor aesthetic quality, but when we're looking for an enhancement we're looking for a much finer aesthetic finish?

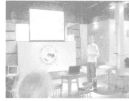

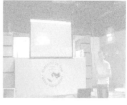

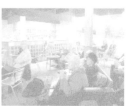

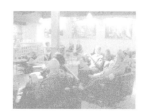

DISCUSSANT
Café Scientifique
Major interventions are something we need to think carefully about if they are not curative. We do need to think carefully about the issue of identity. We are not necessarily as separate from the world as we in the West tend to assume... There are potentials for a downside, whether it's the person's attitude to themselves, or their attitude to other people, if they have non-medical replacements that do literally make them into a hyper being. And what of other people's perceptions of them?

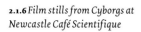

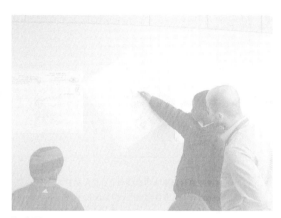

Fig. 2.1.7

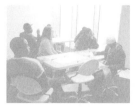

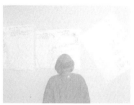

Fig. 2.1.8

Fig. 2.1.9

MY SPACE, MY CITY, MY WORLD

—

STEPHEN LAWRENCE CENTRE

'That time at the Stephen Lawrence Centre – we did that event down there, and some of the questions that came out were quite left-field and not the sort you get at a peer review conference, for example. It was worthwhile and interesting to have to think about those, because when you're working in a particular field you have your agreed norms, and it's very easy to stay in your comfort zone and not have those norms queried or challenged.'

TONY CASS
Institute of Biomedical Engineering,
Imperial College London

'The conference aims to build young people's confidence in making their voices heard in the places where decisions are made about design, engineering, economics and the future.'

IGNITE!, MY SPACE, MY CITY, MY WORLD
Conference report

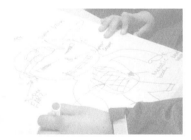

Fig. 2.1.10

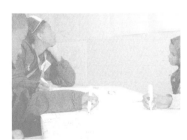

Fig. 2.1.11

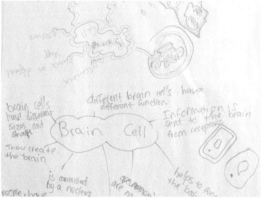

Fig. 2.1.12

2.1.7 – 2.1.11 *Designing cyborgs at the Stephen Lawrence Centre*
2.1.12 *Detail of a system controlled by brain cells*

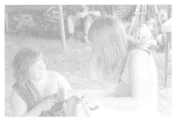

Fig. 2.1.13

Fig. 2.1.14

GUERRILLA
SCIENCE CAMP
—
SECRET GARDEN
FESTIVAL

GUERRILLA SCIENCE CAMP
Because Truth Is Stranger Than Fiction
'We know, we know – you think science is boring. But don't let the uninspired teachers you had ruin it for you. Science isn't about reducing life's complexity to humdrum mundanities – it is about how spectacularly amazing reality is. Let us assault your senses, open your eyes and blow your mind. Discover why you might already have a mind-bending parasite lodged in your brain, listen to the music of the stars, and learn to shoot flames with custard powder in our chemistry kitchen.'
GUERRILLA SCIENCE CAMP
Event handout

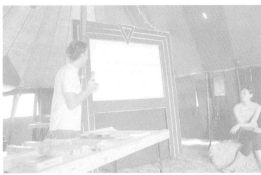

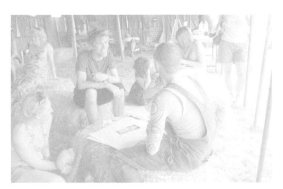

Fig. 2.1.15

Fig. 2.1.16

2.1.13 – 2.1.16 *Combining bodies with products at the Guerilla Science Tent*
2.1.17 *Secret Garden Festival bingo session*
2.1.18 *Secret Garden Festival grounds*

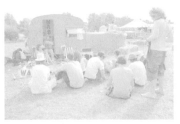

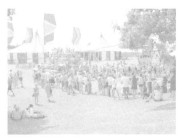

Fig. 2.1.17

Fig. 2.1.18

2.2

TECHNO BODIES; HYBRID LIFE?

Material Beliefs curated *Techno Bodies; Hybrid Life?*, an evening of discussion and debate at London's Dana Centre, part of the Science Museum.

All four collaborations contributed to the sessions, combining the researchers' descriptions of their work with social questions posed by the designers. Framing the research in this way encouraged participants to offer their own views about the ethics and effects of these technologies.

These contributions helped to shape the collaborations by providing alternative perspectives to fuel design concepts.

'Look at all these people in the same room: medics, engineers, designers, creative thinkers and heavyweight technical people. It's really exciting that they are talking to each other.'

AUDIENCE MEMBER
Techno Bodies; Hybrid Life? at the Dana Centre, Science Museum

'There should be a way in which culture can feed back into the applications of technology, because at the moment we are given something – we've got the internet, we've got telephones, we've got televisions, we've got thousands of cars, we've got hair dryers, DIY stuff – and nobody's asked us what we think about it. This is why engineers and designers should be dealing with public engagement all the time. They should be testing their ideas out on people and exposing themselves freely so that people can interrogate them – those who can be bothered.'

JIMMY LOIZEAU
Department of Design, Goldsmiths

TECHNO BODIES; HYBRID LIFE?

—

DANA CENTRE

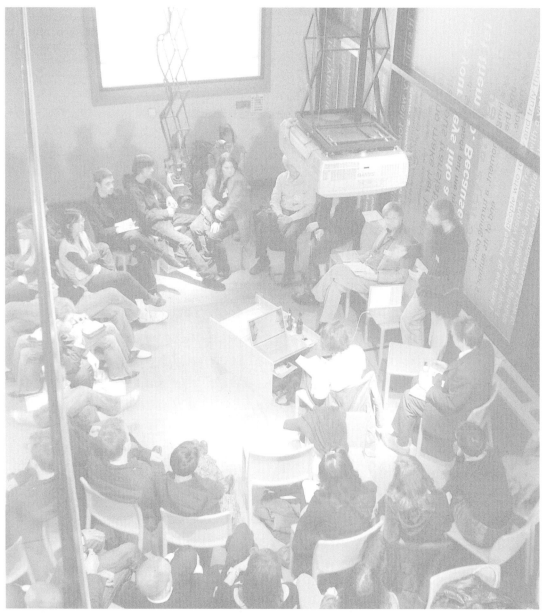

Fig. 2.2.1

Meet engineers, designers and thinkers who are blurring boundaries between technologies and your body. What counts as a hybrid life form and how might it affect you?

Contributors from the Bristol Robotics Laboratory, the Future of Humanity Institute at Oxford University, the Institute of Biomedical Engineering at Imperial College London and University of Reading's Cybernetics group will present ongoing projects for your delectation in this evening of demonstration and discussion.

Highlights include the chance to meet EcoBot – a fly-eating robot whose digestive juices power-up microbial fuel cells to generate it's own power. Hear about a robot controlled by a culture of neural cells via a wireless link. Will the biological features of our future appliances make them more like pets? We'll also be discussing the technologies helping us to live longer – is it sustainable to mend and replace our frail bodies? Finally, consider how tiny sensors in the digital plaster could use your mobile phone to tell you to slow down. And what about sharing this information – how might this body network connect to the internet, will we be monitoring each other's activity?

If all this whets your appetite for further involvement, ask the Material Beliefs team what roles you could play in their ongoing project. Have your say as we discuss these new hybrids: are we becoming our own products?

The Dana Centre, Tuesday 22 January 2008, 19:00 – 20:30

AMIR EFTEKHAR, *Researcher, Institute of Biomedical Engineering*
TOBIE KERRIDGE, *Designer, Goldsmiths*
NICK OLIVER, *Researcher, Institute of Biomedical Engineering*

JAMES AUGER, *Designer, Royal College of Art*
JIMMY LOIZEAU, *Designer, Goldsmiths*
ALAN WINFIELD, *Engineer, Bristol Robotics Laboratory*

ELIO CACCAVALE, *Designer, Goldsmiths*
JULIA DOWNES, *Researcher, Reading Cybernetics*
MARK HAMMOND, *Researcher, Reading Pharmacy / Cybernetics*
DIMITRIS XYDAS, *Researcher, Reading Cybernetics*

AUBREY DE GREY, *Chairman and Chief Science Officer, Methuselah Foundation*
ANDERS SANDBERG, *Neuroscientist, Future of Humanity Institute*
SUSANA SOARES, *Designer, Goldsmiths*

Fig. 2.2.2

2.2.1 *Aubrey de Grey in discussion at the Dana event*
2.2.2 *Dana Centre press release*
2.2.3 – 2.2.6 *Participants, Techno Bodies; Hybrid Life?*

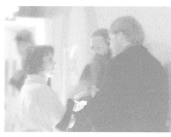

Fig. 2.2.3

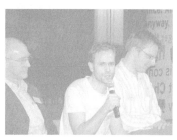

Fig. 2.2.4

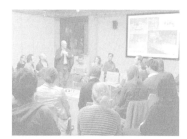

Fig. 2.2.5

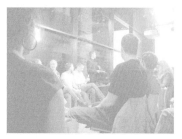

Fig. 2.2.6

Fig. 2.2.7

DIGITAL PLASTER

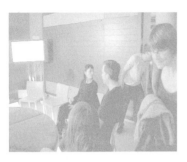

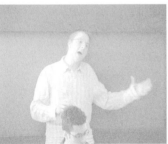

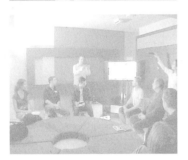

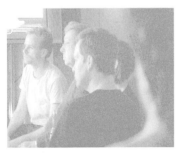

CONVERSATIONS AT THE DANA CENTRE

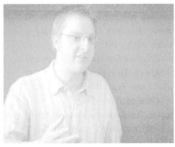

NICK
This is a platform to measure heart rate, accelerometer data, respiratory rate, your oxygen saturation in your blood and even metabolic things like glucose and fats in your blood, and if you view this as a non-invasive platform for sensing then it's one step towards personalised healthcare... Your mobile phone could call me at 3 a.m. to let me know you've had an unusual heart rhythm, or it could call you to ask if you are OK.

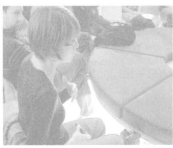

PARTICIPANT
I came along to this because I'm a diabetic, and I'm really interested in this area because I've already got a kind of prototype, an insulin pump. It's a very modern one. It shows me in real time what my sugar level is doing.

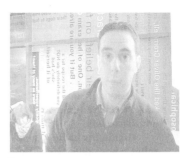

PARTICIPANT
I have to say, the technology is advancing, but I was disappointed that the discussion was about the design and aesthetics and not about the different aspects of healthcare that this could help.

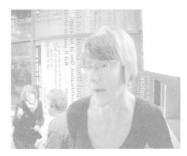

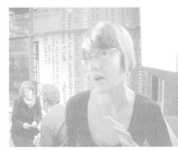

PARTICIPANT
I was very interested in the Digital Plaster session, looking at how you could wear devices that would give you feedback about what your body is doing, which is helpful in the medical context, both for the person who is wearing it but potentially for other people who are trying to help you improve your health.

Fig. 2.2.8

ECOBOT

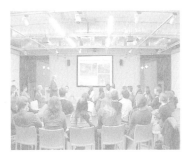

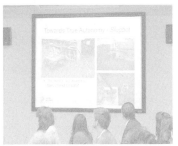

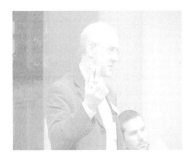

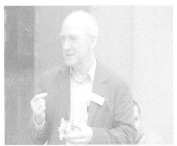

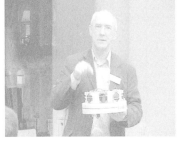

ALAN

We're going to be talking about robots that eat food. You may think: what's the point of robots that eat food? Well, the point is this. If in the future robots are going to be really useful, rather than just experiments in the lab, they are going to have to fend for themselves. A lot of roboticists worry about intelligence, AI – robots knowing what to do next. In our lab we are interested in a different kind of autonomy – energy autonomy. So I'm going to talk about a series of robots: a slugbot, a fly-eating robot, and the world's first robot with an artificial digestive system.

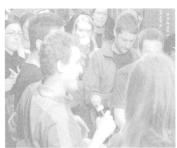

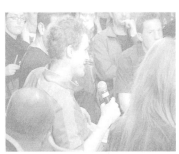

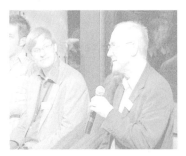

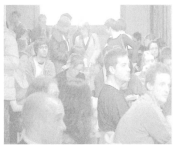

PARTICIPANT

Are we anywhere near the point where we start to feel guilty or bad about turning these sorts of hybrid machines off?

ALAN

Rest assured that we are a long, long, long way from even beginning to build what we might think would be artificial consciousness. But if we believed we could build it – which we don't at the moment – then I agree with you, we would have to worry about the ethical question of whether we'd switch it on or not.

2.2.7 – 2.2.8 *Film stills from Techno Bodies; Hybrid Life? at the Dana Centre*

Fig. 2.2.9

LIFE EXTENSION

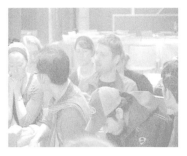

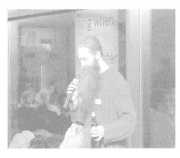

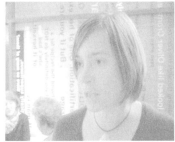

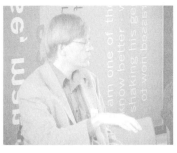

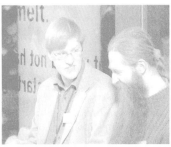

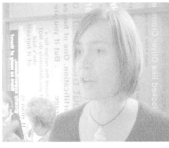

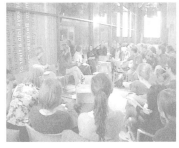

PARTICIPANT

As a human race we're part of an ecosystem, and so if we prolong life to the point where people can live indefinitely, then the population will rise and rise and eventually we'll run out of resources. I don't see a way that extending life will be sustainable in the long term, unless people decide to stop reproducing. It's hard enough to get people to agree on writing off Third World debt, so to make people all over the world consume differently – I don't think it's realistic.

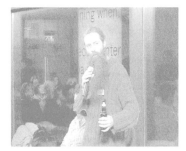

AUBREY

If we were actually able to defeat ageing, then everything would change, and so it's something that is relevant to every creative discipline.

Fig. 2.2.10

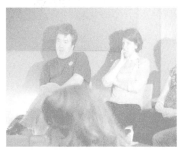

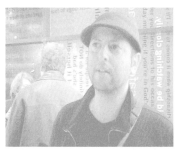

ANIMAT

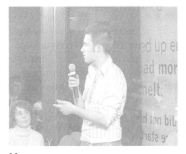

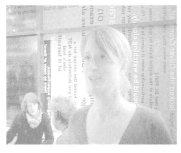

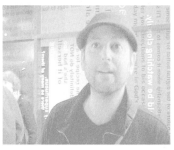

MARK

We're a collaboration between cybernetics and pharmacy, and we're working on embodying a culture of neural cells using a robot to basically give it a body. This allows us to see the whole brain at once, and we can study how the interactions between those cells result in the behaviour that we see. This is a new paradigm – in current neuroscience methods you can only study perhaps a small part of the brain at once, whereas we can study the whole brain and its relationship to behaviour and processing.

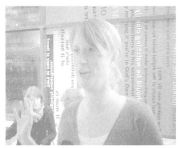

PARTICIPANT

I admire the fact that these guys are challenging contemporary scenarios. Sometimes you have issues of ethics and fears, and they managed to capture a few interesting scenarios. In general, I think that design is a strategy for questioning culture... and I think these guys are questioning culture and generating new scenarios.

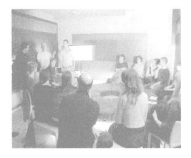

2.2.9 – 2.2.10 *Film stills from Techno Bodies; Hybrid Life? at the Dana Centre*

2.3

ROYAL COLLEGE
OF ART
DESIGN INTERACTIONS
—
THE BIOTECH
PROJECT

Material Beliefs set up a four-week project for Royal College of Art students in the Design Interactions course. The aim was to connect designers' fascination with, and trepidation about, biotechnology with a mundane and situated understanding of lab-based research, along with an awareness of contemporary issues in science and society at large.

Researchers at the Institute of Biomedical Engineering and University of Reading took up visiting tutor roles at the RCA, providing feedback on the student's work. A selection of this work was included in *Human Futures*, a book published by the Foundation for Art and Creative Technology (FACT).

'It was only when Nelly came in with her scattering of porcelain objects and said to me, "What do these mean to you?" that I said to myself, "Oh my God, I'll have to start thinking differently now!"'.

OLIVE MURPHY
*Institute of Biomedical Engineering, Imperial College London
on her collaboration with Nelly Ben Hayoun, Design Interactions, Royal College of Art*

SCIENCE AND SOCIETY

As sites for collaboration between engineers, chemists, biologists, administrators and medics, biomedical engineering labs are spaces for the production of new technologies, which bring together soft tissues and silicon, to heal and enhance the functions of bodies.

How can designers situate this research into broader society? By setting up interventions with engineers and scientists, along with publics, bioethicists and sociologists, design can create products, services and events which stage sophisticated conversations, by plotting original paths through this cross-disciplinary space.

Design can offer more than a critique of biomedical engineering, it can devise speculative methods for embedding science into society. For this project you are asked to take on a hypothetical role at the Institute of Biomedical Engineering, as a designer in residence, taking emerging technologies into non-medical contexts.

You will identify a technological focus to respond to, drawing upon your experiences at the workshop, other research activities at IBE, or other institutes for biomedical engineering.

You might consider...
· Hypothetical lifestyle products which explore the transition from medical applications into a broader consumer space
· Building design objects that take on bioethical or philosophical concerns
· How to facilitate a discussion about biomedical engineering technologies with non specialist audiences
· The role of design documentation as a way of capturing and inscribing scientific processes and protocols

WEEK 1 – WORKSHOP & DISCUSSION
Tuesday 22 April — Student workshop at IBE, briefing
Wednesday 23 April — Round table discussion with Elio and Tobie
Wednesday 23 April — Evening talk – Paul Thurston (Think Public)

WEEK 2 – TUTORIALS & RESEARCH
Monday 28 April — Tutorials Elio & Tobie
Tuesday 29 April — Tutorials Elio & Tobie
Thursday 1 May — Evening talk – Tom Shakespeare (PEALS)

WEEK 3 – TUTORIALS & DESIGN
Thursday 8 May — Mark (University of Reading) & Elio, Patrick (IBE) & Tobie
Thursday 8 May — Evening talk – Alex Wilkie (Goldsmiths)

WEEK 4 – TUTORIALS & CRIT
Monday 12 May — Round table discussion with Elio and Tobie
Thursday 12 May — Crit

THE BRIEF

Fig. 2.3.I

2.3.1 *Brief for the Science and Society project*

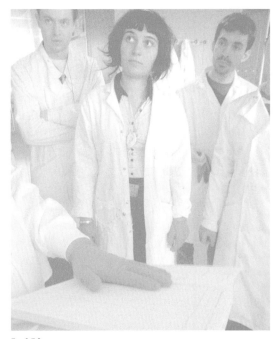

Fig. 2.3.2

The four-week project started with a two-day workshop at the Institute of Biomedical Engineering. The aim of the workshop was to provide those from the RCA with an embedded view of biomedical technologies, and for those based at IBE to have a fresh set of responses to their research.

IBE
LAB VISIT

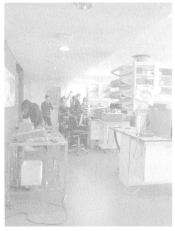

Fig. 2.3.3

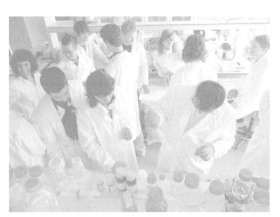

Fig. 2.3.4

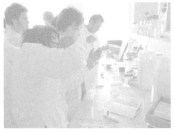

Fig. 2.3.5

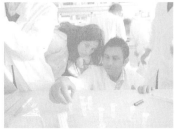

Fig. 2.3.6

2.3.2 – 2.3.2 *A lab tour at the Institute of Biomedical Engineering*
2.3.4 – 2.3.6 *Extracting DNA from cheek cells*

TUTORIAL WITH AUSTIN

Fig. 2.3.7

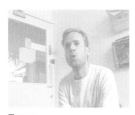

TOBIE

Two and half weeks into a four-week project, I've been meeting the students with Patrick. Patrick is a researcher at IBE and a lecturer there, and what we are trying to do with that is encourage the students to talk to different audiences about their work so it's less of a kind of internal situation, and they're not just having these conversations with themselves and doing fantastic designs, but they are also, in a way, accountable to Patrick, whose perspective encompasses a different set of issues. So by doing these joint tutorials we are trying to extend the students' experience and get them thinking in different ways.

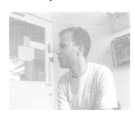

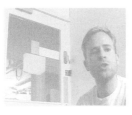

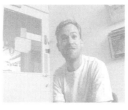

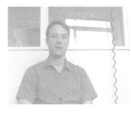

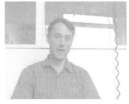

PATRICK

My contribution here is on the technical side, and I can also come in on the ethical side of things. So from this perspective I can add to their viewpoint. I got the impression that a lot of the projects were design led, with some of the ethical and technical issues needing development.

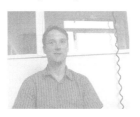

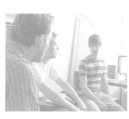

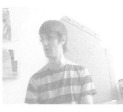

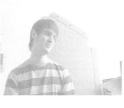

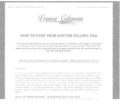

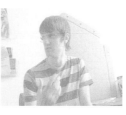

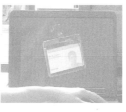

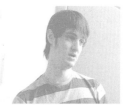

AUSTIN

My initial idea is to create an orexin reactive ID badge, which senses and displays biometric data about the doctors' wellbeing. The pressure on doctors and medical staff within hospitals to perform their duties to the highest standard is immense. As new government targets and incentives are designed to give the patient better healthcare, they inevitably place more pressure on the medical staff – which worsens their overall health. Stressed and tired medical staff will inevitably deliver poor medical care to the patients, so new cost-effective biotechnologies have been employed to monitor the doctor and feed relevant information about their health to the patient.

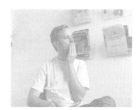

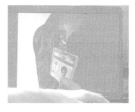

2.3.7 *Film stills from Royal College of Art tutorial*

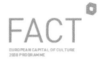

humanfutures

12 May, 2008.

Dear Colleague,

We are writing to invite your contribution to an exciting new book titled '**Human Futures**', which will be published in October/November 2008 alongside the BBC Radio 3 Free Thinking festival in Liverpool. The book will be a high-quality, design-led publication featuring scholarly essays, graphics, creative writing and innovative page layouts.

The themes of the book are structured around the Human Futures programme at the Foundation for Art and Creative Technology (FACT) in Liverpool, which has brought leading artists, philosophers, designers and scientists to debate this broad subject area. Human Futures is FACT's flagship programme during Liverpool's year as European Capital of Culture. Our publisher is Liverpool University Press, which is the exclusive contractor for FACT's publications. We have a dynamic team of producers that will work to turn this book around within a very short time frame. An integral part of this approach is to access essays that authors are already working on and are near completion, but which have yet to find a home. We welcome proposals for any type of submission but are particularly interested in publishing quirky pieces from established authors who might not typically publish such material.

We wonder what you could submit that is less traditionally academic, but which speaks to themes of your work on human futures. It need not be something like this; a more traditional essay, short or long would also appeal. However, we want to see what we can uncover that is unusual, different and original. Alternatively, you might submit to us text from newspaper interviews that never made it passed the editorial desk or an audio-visual form of a presentation, from which we could utilize the text. Other ideas include short stories, an Epilogue to a recent book or Prologue to a project about to be conceived/published, written in a more personal format, or a handwritten memoir/reflection. It's a really openly defined project, so let us know what might appeal.

With this in mind, the more difficult news is that our **copy deadline is 9 June for receipt of your contribution**. We ask you to consider carefully your capacity to meet this deadline before proposing a contribution, as we are working with a publisher deadline of 30 June for all edited copy. However, we do stress that this will be a novel and exciting book, reaching new audiences and bringing together previously isolated points of view. For this reason, we hope you might welcome this opportunity to be a part of it. To summarize, for written matter, we can receive any of the following: long essays (5,000 words), short essays (2,000 words), creative writing (3,000 words), original quotes responding to our brief (see below for key questions) and audio/visual matter.

If you would like more information about the FACT programme, please see the related website below. For more details on the book, please see the synopsis below. For correspondence, please contact us at email@andymiah.net Finally, to get a better sense of the Human Futures programme, please take a look at the website below.

Yours Sincerely,

Dr Andy Miah, Professor Mike Stubbs & Ms Laura Sillars
Editors of Human Futures.
http://humanfutures.fact.co.uk

Fig. 2.3.8 *Invite to submit content to Human Futures book*

HUMAN FUTURES

BOOK

MATERIAL BELIEFS

Shahid Aziz, Elio Caccavale, Tony Cass, Patrick Degenaar, Rob Fenton, Tobie Kerridge, Thao Le, Olive Murphy and Nick Oliver, with Cathrine Kramer, Nelly Ben Hayoun, Will Carey, Daisy Ginsberg and Sascha Pohflepp

What we've got much better at doing, is understanding how to make biology and electronics talk together. The idea a few years ago of having a biological silicon hybrid was science fiction, but now because silicon technologies are getting smaller, and our understanding of the organisation of biological systems is getting better, one can see how you can put the two together (Tony Cass, Institute of Biomedical Engineering).

How can designers situate this research into broader society? By setting up interventions with engineers and scientists, along with publics, bioethicists and sociologists, design can create products, services and events which stage sophisticated conversations, by plotting original paths through this cross-disciplinary space.

Taking the biological silicon hybrids under development at Institute of Biomedical Engineering as a start point – the electronic prosthetics, implanted sensors, biometric data and wireless body networks – how would designers situate biomedical engineering within everyday near futures? The following projects reference the playful reconstitution of these engineered systems within more tactical and personal formats including the familial relationships with machines, faking biometric data, bioprospecting, medicating laughter and healthy films.

Material Beliefs ran a four week brief with postgraduate students from Design Interactions at the Royal College of Art. The project launched with a workshop at the Institute of Biomedical Engineering, encouraging students to respond to emerging biotechnology applications. Outcomes depicted in the following pages included a range of speculative products and services that situated technoscience research within an everyday context. As such, they explored mundane, idiosyncratic, or domestic contexts of use.

2.3.9 *Description of Material Beliefs contribution to Human Futures book*

Fig. 2.3.9

STUDENT PROJECTS
FOR HUMAN
FUTURES BOOK

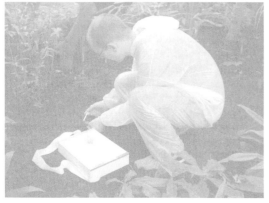

Fig. 2.3.10

Fig. 2.3.11

PROSPECT RESORT
Sascha Pohflepp

Bioprospecting describes the practice of collecting plant and animal life for pharmaceutical research, potentially leading to the development of novel medicines. Despite associations with colonialism, bioprospecting has recently been linked to synthetic biology, and the various efforts of collecting and sequencing the genomes of a vast number of organisms.

Facilitated by the participatory culture of the internet, biological research is becoming more accessible and affordable. The amateur bioprospector returns his or her findings to a lively community, much like amateur astronomers. Unlike in astronomy, those who dive into the subject will often have a personal investment in their activities. Many bioprospectors might be suffering from a degenerative disease like ALS or Parkinson's and may want to actively participate in the search for a cure while their illness progresses.

Prospect Resort is a fictional hotel in South America which provides these personal bioprospectors with a base for their ventures into the Amazon rainforest. Being hotel, high-grade laboratory and hospital in equal parts, it would be ideally located in one of the most biodiverse ecosystems of the planet. Often accompanied by their families, residents search for specimens of rare plants and animals that have shown promising results in earlier research. The prospector's equipment consists of a portable sterile laboratory cabinet and simple tools to take tissue samples with. Additionally, a small local economy has also developed around the resort, with stalls offering biopsies of small animals and plants from inaccessible areas in the forest.

Prospect Resort suggests a form of contemporary colonialism, where its services are aimed at the future needs of the wealthy. Despite this, it also traces a perceived shift in popular culture towards amateur participation in the production of medical information. Perhaps there will be a real opportunity for individuals to participate in genetic research in the near future, possibly even with the support of the public health system.

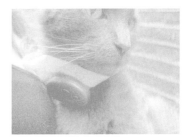

Fig. 2.3.14

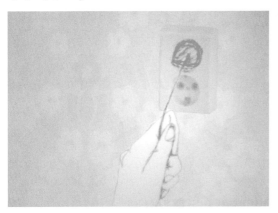

Fig. 2.3.12

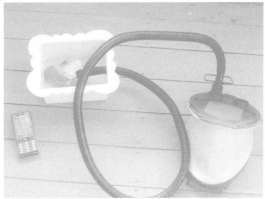

Fig. 2.3.15

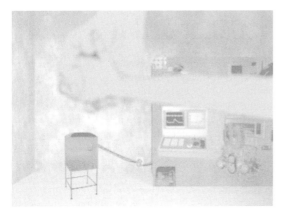

Fig. 2.3.13

HEART
Cathrine Kramer

Heart is an animation which explores the end of life. The story situates biomedical technologies in the home, where a machine is extending the life of the main character's terminally ill mother. Rather than being an effect of illness, the final event of death now follows the cessation of the machine. When is it time to pull the plug?

The animation shows how as a result of dependent relationships between humans and machines, it is no longer clear what constitutes a person. Is it possible for the girl to maintain a relationship with just the vital signs of her mother's heart? To what extent do the behaviours and functions of the machine contribute to this bond?

Heart explores the familial contexts for biomedicine and end of life, and shows how echoes of these relationships continue in the devices which supported a loved one, even after the plug has been pulled.

CATHY THE HACKER
Nelly Ben Hayoun

In this short film, the central character Cathy is compelled to wear a biometric monitor. It broadcasts a stream of data to an unseen agency – this could be an insurance company with vested interest in Cathy's health, or a medical institution implementing a service designed to extend the life-spans of it's users. Either way, the function of the implant contrives an intrusion upon Cathy's life. It erodes her personal freedom, enforcing a structure tailored for the production of the right 'kind' of biometric information.

So Cathy devises a series of elaborate deceits, allowing her go out with friends, or just put her feet up, while still providing optimal data. A three legged cat is coaxed into wearing the device, hopping around the flat to generate fake activity. The closing spin cycle of the washing machine also does a good job. Cathy then skillfully disassembles the device and links it to a foot pump, to be reluctantly operated by her daughter.

These sequences are interrupted with footage from a conversation with Olive Murphy, a researcher at the IBE. Olive speculates how data generated by the sensing devices developed through her own research (an implantable blood pressure monitor) might be circumvented. 'Once it's implanted it's always there' explains Olive, and we follow Cathy into a lift where she rests, to prevent transmission of her data.

2.3.16 *Homegrown*
2.3.17 *Microbe Controllers*

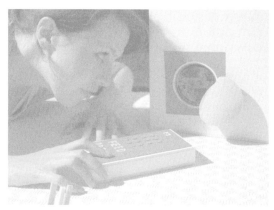

Fig. 2.3.17

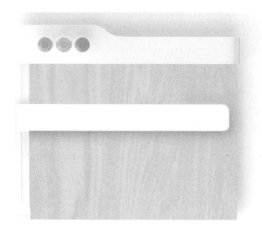

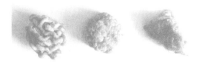

Fig. 2.3.16

HOMEGROWN
Will Carey

Sourcing local foods and keeping livestock have recently been portrayed as qualitative experiences. Though this invigorated appetite for foraging and rearing comes at a premium to shopping for food at a supermarket, this is about investing personal effort over a long period of time, in order to gain the freshest produce.

Homegrown began as an exploration of how the domestic production of vitro meat might sit within this context. How would cell culturing leave the laboratory and enter the home? Would methods of production at such small scales enable meat to be treated as a material, combining cells derived from a range of animals, creating compound or hybrid foods with unexpected textures and flavours? Scenarios were developed to suggest new aesthetics for food production, and novel rituals for preparing and tasting in vitro meats.

MICROBE CONTROLLERS:
BIOLOGICAL LANDSCAPING AT HOME
Daisy Ginsberg

Microbes are the enemy. We spend millions on anti-bacterial products, fearing the microbes in our food, in our homes, on our hands. Yet with microbes in our body outnumbering our own cells, they might have more to offer than we thought. *Escherichia coli* – or *E.coli* – is the workhorse of the biotech lab and the model bacterium, having played a key role in the development of many biotechnologies. Easily manipulated and cultured in a laboratory, we probably know more about this lowly bacteria than any other living creature on earth. Craig Venter is fishing the world's oceans, assembling a vast library of diverse microbes, prospecting for new strings of genetic code that may yield new and profitable commercial applications. Microbes are being genetically engineered to create biological computers, infiltrating the previously grey technology of silicon with a new green dimension.

Microbe Controllers considers a domestic landscape where microbes and other engineered microscopic organisms are cultivated to perform useful tasks in the home. Aware of this microscopic horticultural landscape living alongside us, will our attitudes to what we accord 'living' status change? What are the ethical issues in making living, disposable consumer products? Are we economically compelled to develop biotechnologies and consider the ethics later? At what scale do we value life? In the lab, bacteria, neurons and other cellular scale 'things' are not attributed 'living' status, but as the size and complexity increases, we begin to feel tenderness or anxiety.

Should we be fighting for microbe rights? Cemeteries and memorials for dead kettles and expired lab cultures? Microbes may not have feelings – as far as we understand – but perhaps we should we explore the ethics of enslaving them before the Argos catalogue is filled with living electronics.

Chapter 3

THE NEUROSCOPE AND OTHER FUTURE SHOCKS

—

DEVELOPING DESIGNS

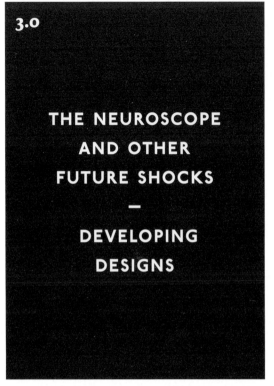

3.0

THE NEUROSCOPE
AND OTHER
FUTURE SHOCKS
—
DEVELOPING
DESIGNS

'Critical design can utilise props, newspaper articles and other means to entice and coax the audience into the discussion. Video, for example, has the ability to operate on the borders between fiction and reality, allowing the audience to enter a parallel world that provides an aperture on possibility.'

JAMES AUGER
Design Interactions, Royal College of Art

'This robot will be the first to have a biological brain.'

KEVIN WARWICK
University of Reading, in conversation with Elio Caccavale and Tobie Kerridge, Interaction Research Studio, Goldsmiths

'Critical design' is a term coined by Tony Dunne (in his book *Hertzian Tales*), who discusses his approach to design in this chapter. Other designers with similar approaches use phrases such as 'speculative design' or 'reflective design' to describe their work. What they all have in common is that they use design to provoke questions about the social implications of new technologies. In doing so, they often blur the boundaries between fact and fiction, between science and art, and between commercial design and academic studies.

You could say that it is essentially a playful approach to design, but also one that takes the future very seriously. This combination of playfulness and seriousness is slippery, in intent and effect – it's hard to define. And so it provokes questions about the role of design itself. What is the 'product' here? Is it an object – the prototype? Is it a process – the research and development, and then dissemination? Or is it perhaps a relationship – the connections made between all those touched by the work?

This chapter traces the evolution of the prototypes developed by the four main design-engineering collaborations in Material Beliefs. Things didn't always go smoothly, chiefly because working methods, and therefore goals and expectations, differed enormously. The designers were primarily on the look-out for meaningful 'narratives' in which to situate novel products; the engineers were more concerned with the transition from scientific theory to physical fact – with making things function.

When these two types of creative problem-solving meshed, however, it was as if a small window opened on to the future – or rather, on to a future. By regarding a design prototype as if it were an actual product or system, you receive a glimpse of a potential world: the world in which such a thing could exist. It's like a small moment of future shock, except that, instead of the future overtaking you, it is you that overtakes the future.

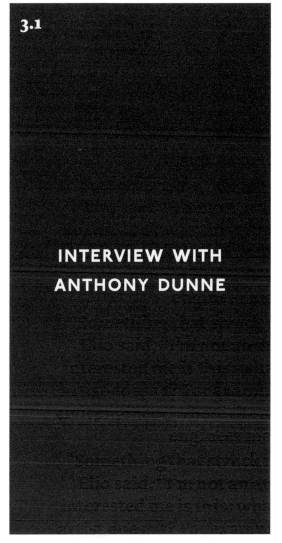

3.1

INTERVIEW WITH ANTHONY DUNNE

The designers in Material Beliefs have at times found it tricky to talk about a type of design that sits somewhere between bio-art (or sci-art) and product innovation. What is distinctive about the type of design that excites you? How do you make a case for it?

I'm interested in design that offers alternatives and makes us think, that acts as a medium to investigate a subject, probe our beliefs and values, challenge our assumptions, and encourage us to imagine how things could be different.

This kind of design exists in a very interesting space between problem-solving and commentary. The former tries to change or fix the world while the latter is directed at changing perception, and therefore values and behaviour. The current global crisis is much deeper than a technical one – we cannot just redesign the planet to suit how we live today. We need to rethink how we live, and that means we have to seriously rethink our values.

Most commentary is parasitical. At its worst it simply pokes fun at the situation it is drawing attention to. But when it is done well, by making sophisticated use of design rhetoric, irony and satire, it can be very effective. The kind of design that excites me puts the methods used in commentary to more constructive uses. Design can't save the planet, it can't fix the world, but maybe it can change the way we think. The design I like helps us think differently. We need to redesign our values and attitudes, not the environment.

There isn't really a place for this kind of design right now, so it exists in a sort of parallel design channel. For some this means it's art, for others it's not 'real'. I see it as a form of design fiction, and like other forms of fiction, it's aimed at the imagination and how we think, which in turn can effect how we behave.

You mention bio- and sci-art. It's very important not to get stuck in media-specific ghettos like bio- art/design,

'Something that struck me as interesting was when Elio said, "I'm not an artist. I'm a designer." What interested me is this: what does a designer do that the artist doesn't? For example, is it like an architect and a civil engineer, where the architect does the fluff and the engineer makes it happen?'

DIMITRIS XYDAS
Department of Mechanical Engineering, University College London

or digital art/design, or even interactive art/design. The work needs to stand up by itself when compared to other art/design works.

As for making a case for it, I think the best way is to just do it, and to do it extremely well. I've found that if people are not open to new ideas and approaches then there's no point trying to persuade them. If you can get it out there, through exhibitions and publications, then open-minded people will find it and one thing will lead to another. Well, that's the theory anyway!

James Auger talks about his practice as linking to critical design. It might be good to have some kind of definition. Is this something you feel you can provide? How does critical design relate to the Design Interactions course and the approaches your students take?

Critical Design uses speculative design proposals to ask questions, provoke debate, raise awareness, and explore alternatives. Its opposite is affirmative design design that reinforces the status quo. It rejects the idea that design can only exist in relation to industry and its narrow agenda, and it sets out to explore other ways design can contribute to society. Design can do so much more than help sell products by making them easy to use, sexy and desirable.

Once you reject this narrow role for design you are in a sort of wilderness. Unlike architecture, law, even engineering, design doesn't seem to exist outside a strictly commercial context. Design has a very limited 'social contract' with society that needs to be renegotiated. One of the main aims of critical design is to expand design's potential beyond narrow commercial concerns – to decouple it from industry and explore how it can be put to other uses.

Let's move on to a related term, 'design for debate'. Where did this come from? Is it a form of 'science and society'?

A few years ago I was commissioned by the RCA to write some briefs for their yearly student competition. I was asked to focus on how designers could engage with emerging technologies. One of the most useful roles they could play, it seemed, was to explore the impact these technologies might have on our daily lives if they were to be implemented; to examine possible implications rather than applications. The design proposals that would come out of such investigations would be hypothetical and explore negative as well as positive possibilities. Their aim would be to spark debate about how to achieve technological futures that reflect the complex, troubled people we are, rather than the easily satisfied consumers and users we are supposed to be. As this was quite an unusual role for design, we decided we should be as clear as possible and named the category 'Design for Debate'.

It seems there has been a maturation in Design Interactions in how students take responsibility for the way their ideas interact with related communities – public groups, scientists, sociologists, etc. Can you say something about this?

I think this is true. We've had great feedback from experts and scientists who've met or worked with our students, and as a result, they're getting more opportunities to present and exhibit at non-design conferences and events. I think projects like the one you ran with our students and Imperial College expose them to other practices and value systems, which really helps. Early on, I think people mistakenly thought the projects that looked at the social or political implications of scientific knowledge were critical of scientists and science. This was never the case. The projects do not function as public communication exercises, but neither do they critique scientific advances. They are simply taking exciting scientific discoveries and fast-forwarding to see how they might impact on our daily lives in the near and not so near future. Sometimes the result can be dystopian, but that's more a reflection of human nature and how market-driven values shape the world we live in, than of science itself.

Themes and technologies explored by Material Beliefs have provided opportunities for the ambitions of lobby groups. It's hard enough to cultivate links between design and science, and then there is an additional need to also be cautious – what do you think?

I think once something is out there it takes on a life of it's own. It could be an image, object, text or idea, but there's very little you can do to control its subsequent interpretations, uses and misuses. It's far more frustrating when designers do 'bad' conceptual or critical design as it damages a still developing design approach. By bad, I mean lacking rigour, poorly executed or unoriginal.

What professional roles do you see for your students, the ones involved in these types of practice?

Thinkers and leaders able to turn their thoughts into compelling stories presented through design. They are able to take complex ideas, analyse and make sense of them, and define project spaces that lead to tangible and engaging design outcomes such as scenarios, prototypes, props and videos. I think they make very good explorers. They're able to navigate unchartered territories, map them, and identify new design opportunities.

A question about the skills students should have. An engineer we are working with was interested to see that students' skills included basic prototyping and electronics. What kind of competencies are you encouraging?

Mainly intellectual competencies – for example, thinking through designing. If they can do this it will serve them well for a long time. Practical skills come and go, and once you have some experience, those skills can be outsourced. Successful design careers are built on vision, originality and judgement.

We place a strong emphasis on learning how to figure out what is and what isn't a worthwhile project to work on, and less emphasis on following or mastering a specific process. Students learn how to establish a vision then figure out how to get there. Many of our students are already highly skilled or have previously worked in industry and come to the RCA to be challenged and pushed, intellectually as well as creatively. They have two years to figure out what they want to do and put a folio of work together that will help them take the first steps after graduation. If we focus too much on practical skills, they will eventually be limited by them.

Anthony Dunne
Design Interactions, Royal College of Art
21 February 2009

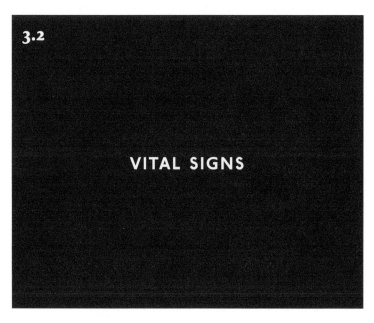

3.2

VITAL SIGNS

The Institute of Biomedical Engineering became a site for interviews, experiments, conversations and workshops. The research and applications being developed there became the subject of student projects, documentary films and a discussion about the future of Type 1 diabetes treatment.

Responding to discussions about surveillance and risk, a set of prototypes were designed. Vital Signs took research into biometric monitoring for chronic health conditions, and repositioned the technology as a system for an anxious parent to monitor their child.

'I think that, previously, the Venn diagrams of the languages that we used and the skill sets that we had would have been miles apart. But they have gradually come together, and now there is this overlap where we speak the same language and have similar ways of thinking. For me, it's mostly been changing the boundaries that we use to describe things.'

NICK OLIVER
Institute of Biomedical Engineering, Imperial College London

'I wasn't one hundred per cent sure what my role or relationship to Material Beliefs was. I think there was a certain amount of 'let's put you together – patient, medic, scientist – and see what happens'. I found the lack of clear role a bit disconcerting to begin with, but came to see it as a journey of discovery. And I enjoyed the journey.'

ROS OAKLEY
Diabetes patient and consultant

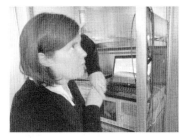

Fig. 3.2.1

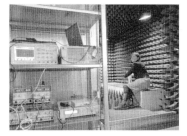

Fig. 3.2.2

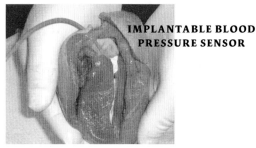

IMPLANTABLE BLOOD PRESSURE SENSOR

Fig. 3.2.3

'...maybe not everybody will want to have one, even if it is for their health. I would have assumed, "Oh, of course this is to everybody's benefit", but you may not want one, you know, people's civil liberties and everything... What if your insurance company will make you have an implant or else won't cover your hospital expenses.'

OLIVE MURPHY
Institute of Biomedical Engineering,
Imperial College London

INTERVIEWS
WITH
RESEARCHERS

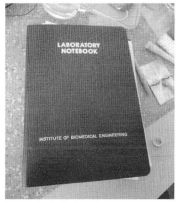

Fig. 3.2.4

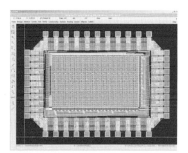

Fig. 3.2.5

3.2.1–3.2.3 *Testing the performance of an implantable sensor*
3.2.4 *Experiments are recorded by date in notebooks*
3.2.5 *Silicon chips are designed using CAD software*
3.2.6 *Tim Constandinou designing a microchip for research, including an bionic eye and an artificial pancreas*
3.2.7 *The manufactured chip is 5mm by 5mm, and is the result of 17 research experiments*

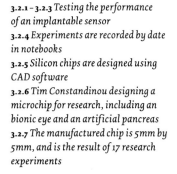

Fig. 3.2.6

BIONIC SILICON CHIP

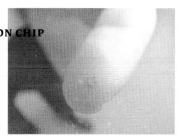

Fig. 3.2.7

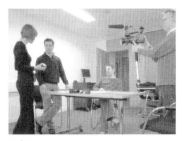

Fig. 3.2.8

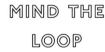

MIND THE

LOOP

Mind the Loop was a filmed conversation between three experts, each with a different understanding of Type 1 diabetes: Ros, a patient with personal insight into managing diabetes; Pantelis, a researcher developing a bionic treatment for the disease; and Nick, a doctor with an interest in diabetes technology research.

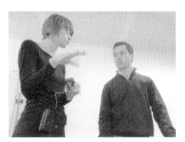

Fig. 3.2.9

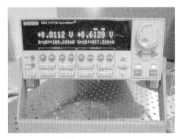

Fig. 3.2.10

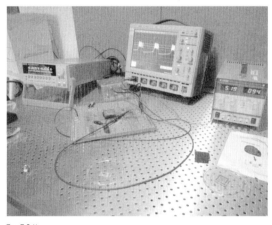

Fig. 3.2.11

'We've looked at the biology of the pancreas and questioned what happens when the pancreas sees glucose and releases insulin, and what we found is that the cells within the pancreas, the beta cells, when they see glucose they do some intelligent algorithm internally and they release insulin. We've taken that function of the beta cell and replicated it using electronic circuits.'

PANTELIS GEORGIOU
*Institute of Biomedical Engineering,
Imperial College London*

'All this data that the technology is capable of producing... There is almost a need for someone to help us with this whole new stream of data that we have. I'm struggling to make sense of it and I'm not sure if the doctors have time to look at it. It's more the data than the physical device that will impact on our relationship.'

ROS OAKLEY
Diabetes patient and consultant

'We imagine that we make technology and that we design things so that they can make our life easier, and our behaviour doesn't need to necessarily change, but actually technology molds us as much as we mould technology'

NICK OLIVER
*Institute of Biomedical Engineering,
Imperial College London*

3.2.8 – 3.2.9 *Steve films the discussion*
3.2.10 *Blood sugar levels are simulated using a voltage signal*
3.2.11 *The voltage signal triggers a pulse that controls insulin release*

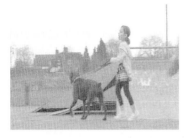

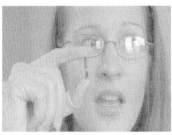

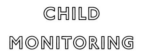

CHILD MONITORING

Discussions with young people revealed their curiosity about how medical technologies move into other contexts of use. Here, the motives for using sensors to monitor the body were discussed, in particular around issues of trust between individuals and institutions, or as a way of managing anxiety.

A documentary, *Cotton Wool Kids*, featured a parent hoping to use a biometric implant to monitor her daughter. The programme revealed how emotive a technology can become when it is subject to individual needs.

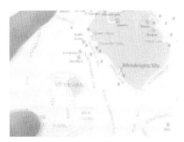

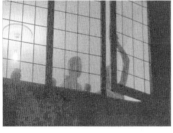

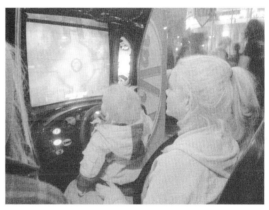

Fig. 3.2.13

Fig. 3.2.12

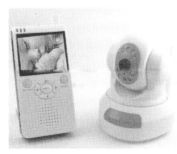

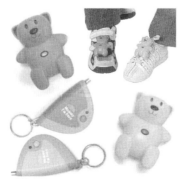

Fig. 3.2.14

Fig. 3.2.15

3.2.12 *A parent discusses an implantable tracking device for her daughter with an engineer, from the documentary Cotton Wool Kids*
3.2.13 *Relationships are mediated by technology*
3.2.14 – 3.2.15 *Products for child monitoring*

VITAL SIGNS
DESCRIPTION

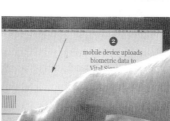

Fig. 3.2.16

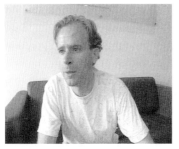

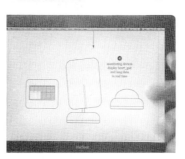

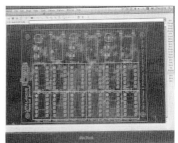

Tobie
I'm interested in how this might move out into other markets – I'm putting it into the context of child monitoring. I'm taking the digital plaster and making a system called Vital Signs, which is a hypothetical but fully working set of prototypes that allow children to be monitored.

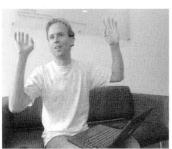

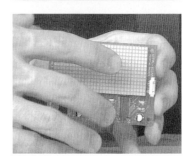

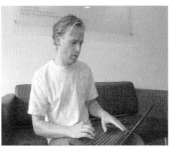

Tobie
Primarily I've been inspired by the digital plaster – an array of body-worn sensors which record biometric data. So you have a sensor on the body that tracks body data and uploads it to a server.

3.2.16 *Film stills from Vital Signs description*

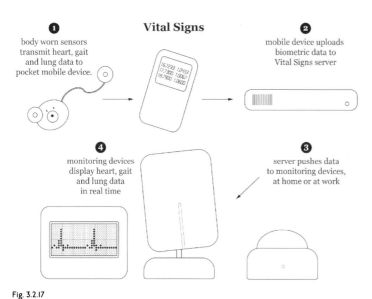

Vital Signs

1 body worn sensors transmit heart, gait and lung data to pocket mobile device.

2 mobile device uploads biometric data to Vital Signs server

4 monitoring devices display heart, gait and lung data in real time

3 server pushes data to monitoring devices, at home or at work

SYSTEMS AND SOFTWARE

Fig. 3.2.17

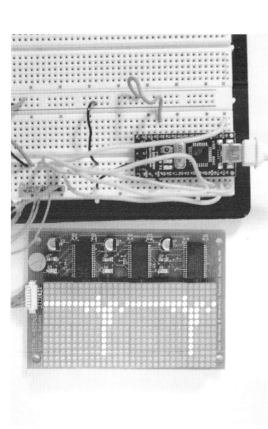

Fig. 3.2.18

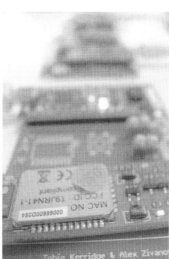

Fig. 3.2.19

3.2.17 *An initial diagram of the system shows three devices that display live biometric data transmitted from the body. The heartbeat is represented in an LED display, footsteps by a display that tilts from left to right, and breathing by the rise and fall of a dome*

3.2.18 – 3.2.19 *The electronics are tested and assembled using custom built modules and off-the-shelf parts. These are USB devices that plug into a PC, and can receive data directly from the PC, or wirelessly from another device using Bluetooth*

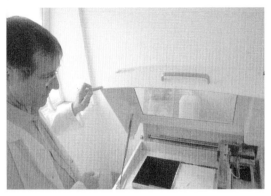

Fig. 3.2.20

Cases for the devices were designed using 3D modelling software. Individual parts were printed using a rapid prototyping machine, initially in plaster to test the form and finally using a plastic material.

MODELLING

AND

FABRICATION

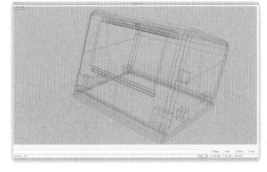

Fig. 3.2.21

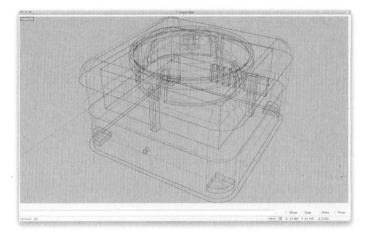

Fig. 3.2.22

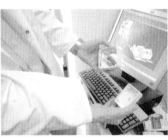

Fig. 3.2.23

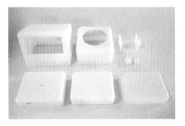

Fig. 3.2.24

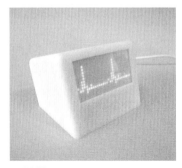

Fig. 3.2.25

MATERIAL BELIEFS
INTERACTION RESEARCH STUDIO

PROTOTYPES
AND
SCENARIO

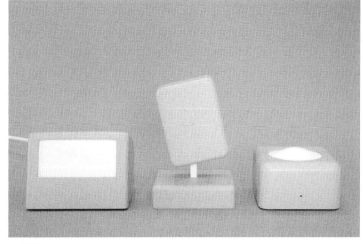

Fig. 3.2.26

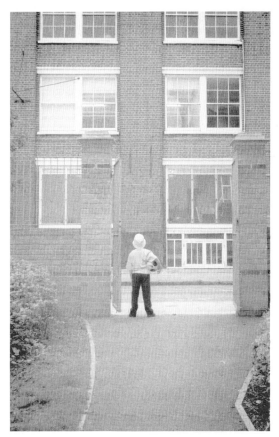

Fig. 3.2.27

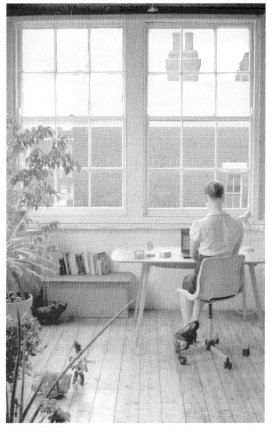

3.2.26 *Finished prototypes*
3.2.27 *Jayden is monitored by Natasja using the Vital Signs devices*

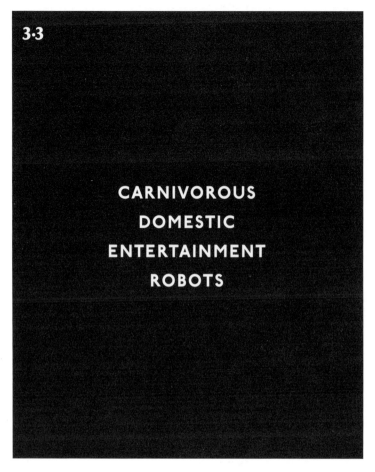

3·3

CARNIVOROUS DOMESTIC ENTERTAINMENT ROBOTS

Carnivorous Domestic Entertainment Robots (CDER) offer an alternative perspective on the development of domestic robots, exploring subtleties of both aesthetics and function that may elicit a symbiotic coexistence with humans in their homes.

Julian Vincent acted as an advisor in the design process. Technological features of CDER take inspiration from Ecobot, an autonomous agent for remote area access developed at Bristol Robotics Laboratory, which uses microbial fuel cells to generate its own power from dead flies. James Auger, Jimmy Loizeau and Aleksandar Zivanovic designed CDER.

'We were manually feeding the fuel cells, so basically it's a case of picking up the dead fly – that had died of natural causes – and dropping it into the chamber of the microbial fuel cell.'

IOANNIS IEROPOULOS
Bristol Robotics Laboratory

'Clearly they don't look like your stereotypical robots. That's something we are very conscious of, and why they exist is also something quite complicated.'

JAMES AUGER
Design Interactions, Royal College of Art

Fig. 3.3.1

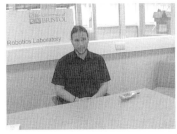

INTERVIEW AT BRISTOL ROBOTICS LAB

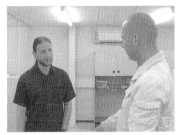

IOANNIS

The main objective of the Ecobot project is energy autonomy for robots. We're interested in developing artificial agents which can extract their energy from the environment. And in doing so, we are employing the microbial fuel cell technology, which uses bacteria to break down organic substrate and produce electricity from that. It's basically a bio-electrochemical transducer.

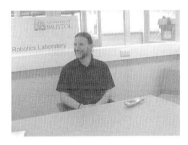

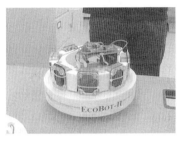

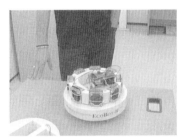

JIMMY

And how much sludge would you say you needed?

IOANNIS

We had eight fuel cells on board. So it was the equivalent of about 200ml of sludge, but that's the catalyst for the reaction, if you like. The fuel for the Ecobot was either dead flies or rotten fruit, and it was operating for 12 days on 8 dead flies.

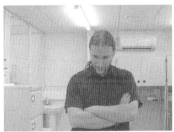

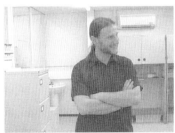

IOANNIS

Ecotbot 2 was a much more powerful robot. We were able to do more with it, so it was able to sense the ambient temperature, process the information, move towards the light, and at the same time communicate information to a base station across the lab. So it had four behvioural tasks out of sludge power.

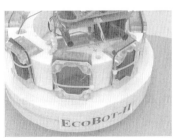

IOANNIS

And then in 2004, two years later, we developed Ecobot 2, which worked with the same bacterial cultures found in sewage sludge, which are capable of breaking down almost anything – that's the good thing about it. But it stinks – that's the bad thing about it.

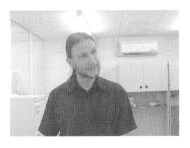

3.3.1 *Ioannis Ieropoulos interviewed at Bristol Robotics Laboratory*

Autonomous agents for remote area access; prototypes developed at Bristol Robotics Laboratory.

BRISTOL ROBOTICS LAB
—
ECOBOT

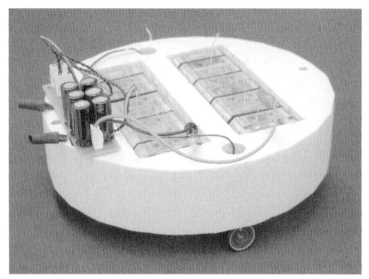

Fig. 3.3.2

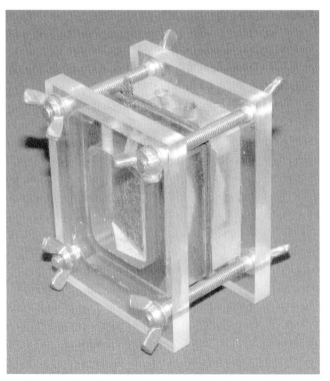

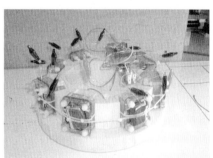

Fig. 3.3.4

Fig. 3.3.3

3.3.2 *EcoBot 1 prototype*
3.3.3 *Microbial fuel cell*
3.3.4 *EcoBot 2 prototype*

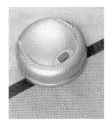

Fig. 3.3.5

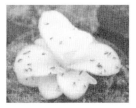

Fig. 3.3.6

CONTEXT FOR DESIGN PROPOSALS

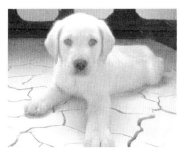

Fig. 3.3.7

'We were thinking initially about ideas around autonomy and what the function of these robots might actually be. Coming from a product design background we are obviously quite in tune with domestic technologies, and we'd seen the Slugbot from Bristol, and this didn't really gel with what we imagined people would want to coexist with. So initially we started thinking about that – what kind of products do we share our lives with? Why we share our lives with them and what they give to us. That was really the starting point.'

JAMES AUGER
Design Interactions, Royal College of Art

'To make them more accessible we've pitched them as entertainment entities, as much as anything, where you're watching these robots attempting to survive through a relationship between animal and machine, so you have two separate entities coming together in a kind of microcosm, similar to a vivarium.'

JIMMY LOIZEAU
Department of Design, Goldsmiths

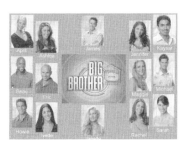

Fig. 3.3.8

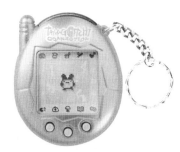

Fig. 3.3.9

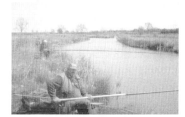

Fig. 3.3.10

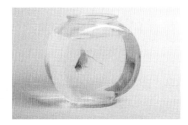

Fig. 3.3.11

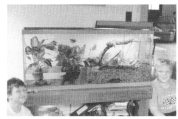

Fig. 3.3.12

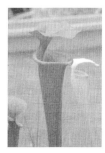

Fig. 3.3.13

3.3.5 – 3.3.13 *Robots could perform a wide range of roles*

SKETCHES

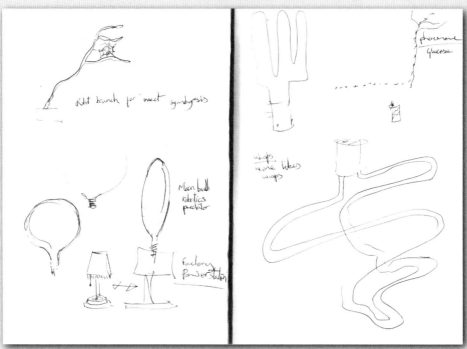

Fig. 3.3.14

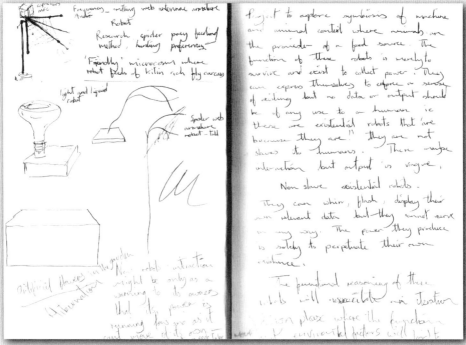

Fig. 3.3.15

3.3.14 – 3.3.17 *Some of Jimmy Loizeau's early sketches for CDER*

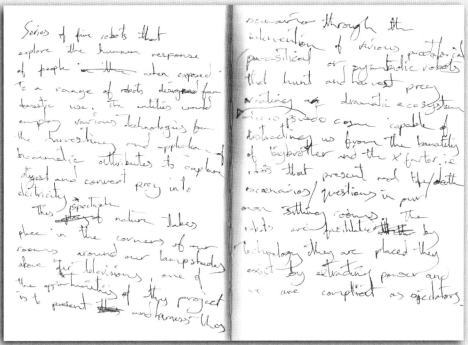

Fig. 3.3.16

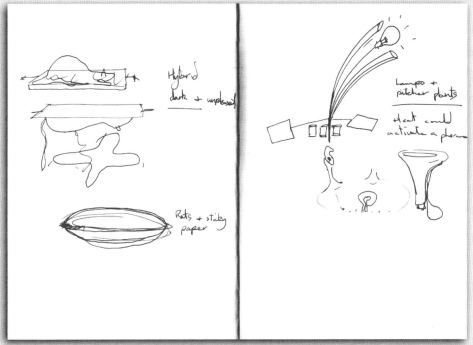

Fig. 3.3.17

INTERVIEW AT THE ROYAL COLLEGE OF ART

Fig. 3.3.18

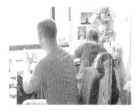

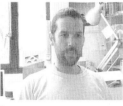

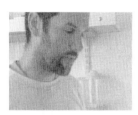

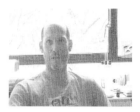

JAMES
There's a family of them – there are five robots – and each of them fulfils a different role. They are a little bit like a colony of ants or bees, where there are different roles and responsibilities for each family member.

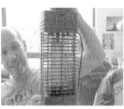

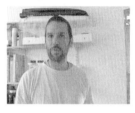

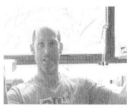

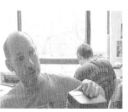

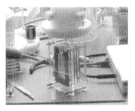

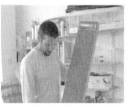

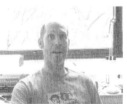

JIMMY
We just coined a new phrase which is 'Robot Robot', or I have, and it's a robot for robots. James doesn't agree with it, he calls it something else. But it's a robot robot and it lives on this [holds up fly catcher]. It basically steals its energy by nicking all the flies from this UV fly killer, and basically it's a slave to other robots. That's why it's a robot robot.

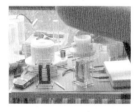

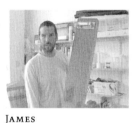

JIMMY
We've also drawn parallels with artificial environments such as Big Brother, Wife Swap and TV programmes like that. We thought why not? Why should the TV be one of the predominant entertainment systems in the house when there are other things like vivariums. And we've got our robots, which do have a function but they could also be entertaining as a spectacle of life and death.

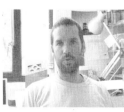

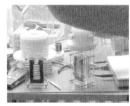

JAMES
A few people have asked us, 'Are these Robots?' 'Why are they robots?' 'They are not robots.' There's not really much agreement, even within the field of robotics, on what a robot is – it's very vague. So what we wanted to do was to take advantage of this vagueness of definition, and say, well yes, they are robots but if we are going to coexist with them, then they have to live within human terms and conditions.

JIMMY
This is a microbial fuel cell, which through a very complicated process of exchange creates electricity from dead flies and moths.

3.3.18 *Film stills from CDER description*

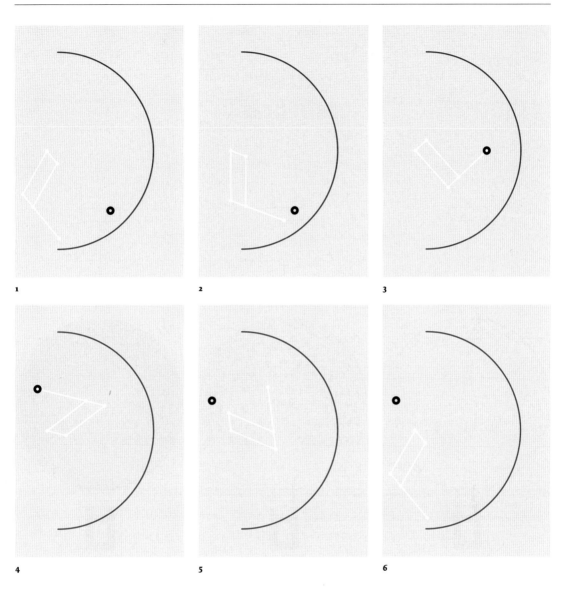

Fig. 3.3.19

ROBOT MOVEMENT

'I've been working on the spider web robot and have written a simulation in Processing. Click anywhere inside the red semicircle to simulate an insect landing on the web (a black circle). The robot moves to grab it, deposits it in a hopper (centre left), then returns to its home position to await another insect.'
ALEKSANDAR ZIVANOVIC
Freelance design engineer

3.3.19 Simulation of robot movement by Aleksander Zivanovic

ROBOT
PROPOSALS

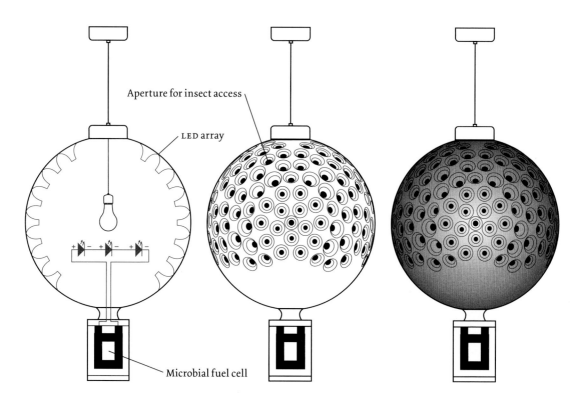

Aperture for insect access

LED array

Microbial fuel cell

Fig. 3.3.20

LAMPSHADE ROBOT

Flies and moths are naturally attracted to light. This lamp shade has holes based on the form of the pitcher plant, enabling access for the insects but no escape. Eventually they expire and fall into the microbial fuel cell underneath. This generates the electricity to power a series of LEDs located at the bottom of the shade. These are activated when the house lights are turned off.

3.3.20 *Lampshade Robot drawing*

MATERIAL BELIEFS
INTERACTION RESEARCH STUDIO

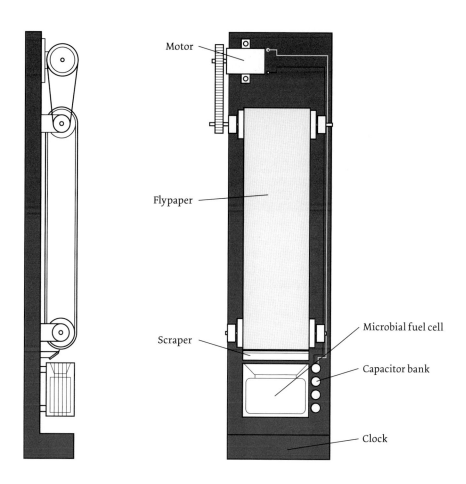

Motor

Flypaper

Scraper

Microbial fuel cell

Capacitor bank

Clock

Fig. 3.3.21

FLYPAPER ROBOTIC CLOCK

This robot uses flypaper as its entrapment mechanism.
This paper is placed on a roller mechanism. At the base of
the roller, a scraper removes any captured insects. These
fall into the microbial fuel cell placed underneath. The
electricity generated by the flies is used to power both a
motor turning the rollers and a small LCD clock.

3.3.21 *Flypaper Robotic Clock drawing*

Armature for building web   Robotic arm fly picker

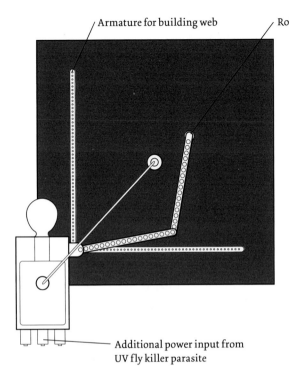

Camera for tracking fly

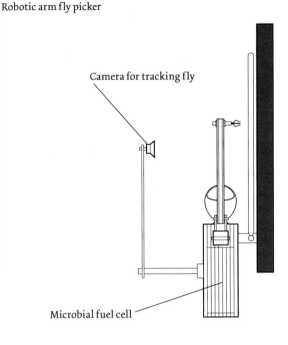

Microbial fuel cell

Additional power input from
UV fly killer parasite

Fig. 3.3.22

FLY-STEALING ROBOT

This robot encourages spiders to build their webs within
its armature. Flies that become trapped in the web are
tracked by a camera. After no movement has been sensed
for ten minutes the robotic arm moves over the dead
fly, picks it up and drops it into the recepticle above the
microbial fuel cell. This generates electricity to partially
power the camera and robotic arm. This robot is not self-
sufficient and relies on the UV fly killer parasite robot to
supplement its energy needs.

UV FLY KILLER PARASITE

A microbial fuel cell is housed underneath an off-the-shelf
UV fly killer. As the flies expire they fall into the fuel cell,
generating electricity that is stored in the capacitor bank.
This energy is available for the fly-stealing robot.

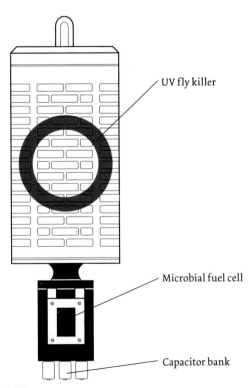

UV fly killer

Microbial fuel cell

Capacitor bank

3.3.22 *Fly-Stealing Robot drawing*
3.3.23 *UV Fly Killer Parasite drawing*

Fig. 3.3.23

MATERIAL BELIEFS
INTERACTION RESEARCH STUDIO

Mechanised iris

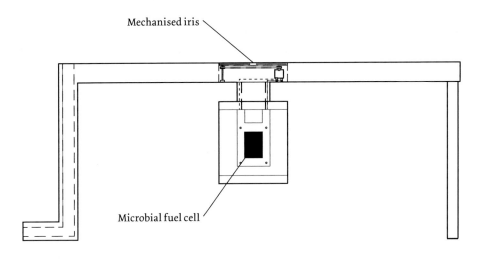

Microbial fuel cell

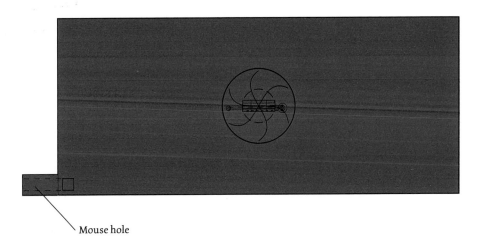

Mouse hole

Fig. 3.3.24

COFFEE TABLE MOUSETRAP ROBOT

A mechanised iris is built into the top of a coffee table.
This is attached to a infra-red motion sensor. Crumbs and
food debris left on the table attract mice, who gain access
to the table top via a hole build into one over size leg. Their
motion activates the iris and the mouse falls into the
microbial fuel cell housed under the table. This generates
the energy to power the iris motor and sensor.

3.3.24 *Coffee table Mousetrap Robot drawing*

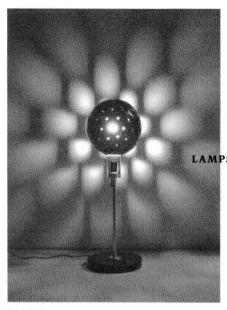

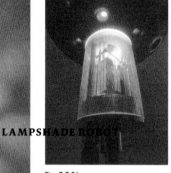

LAMPSHADE ROBOT

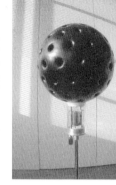

Fig. 3.3.26

Fig. 3.3.27

Fig. 3.3.25

ROBOT
PROTOTYPES

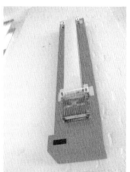
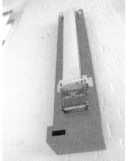

'So as soon as you see a fly coming towards a predatorial robot, which also happens to be a lamp, suddenly the relationship between the fly and the robot lamp becomes charged – and possibly entertaining.'

JIMMY LOIZEAU
Department of Design, Goldsmiths

FLYPAPER ROBOTIC CLOCK

Fig. 3.3.28

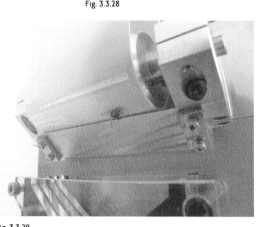

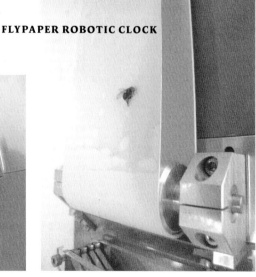

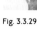

Fig. 3.3.29

Fig. 3.3.30

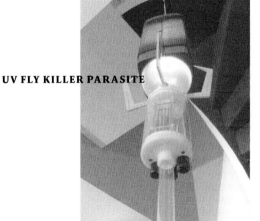

UV FLY KILLER PARASITE

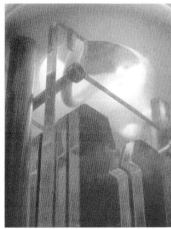

Fig. 3.3.31

Fig. 3.3.32

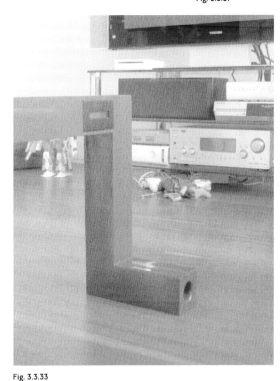

> '**Some of the stories about robots are set in a post-apocalyptic scenario, and actually these robots would survive really nicely in that environment: lots of dead people, lots of flies flourishing. But, there would be no one to entertain, so what would their function be then?**'
> JIMMY LOIZEAU
> *Department of Design, Goldsmiths*

Fig. 3.3.33

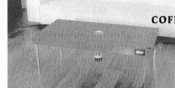

COFFEE TABLE MOUSETRAP ROBOT

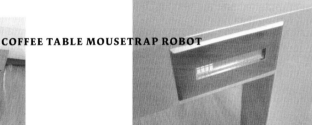

Fig. 3.3.34

Fig. 3.3.35

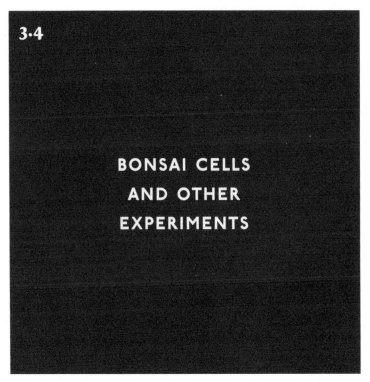

3.4

BONSAI CELLS
AND OTHER
EXPERIMENTS

This project pursued a range of investigative research, taking in life enchantment, the effects of calorie intake on ageing, and stem cell therapies for regenerative medicine.

An interview with Aubrey de Grey led to a discussion about extending life, provoking some design responses that modify the way food is consumed.

A collaboration with the Institute of Ophthamology led to some detailed exploration of the aesthetics of cells. To what extent is it possible to control the pattern and shape of the cell colonies used in regenerative medicine?

'You get used to it and you feel comfortable in an area, and you don't challenge yourself to look at other things. It's almost like you become arrogant. So what I thought was interesting was that they were very open towards someone who was doing a design project and interested in their research...'

'And the other thing was looking at the way they work. It was fascinating to see how they use photography to take pictures of the cells under the microscope. This was quite familiar to me and I thought: how interesting! We probably use almost the same software but with a different purpose.'

SUSANA SOARES
Interaction Research Studio, Goldsmiths

Fig. 3.4.1

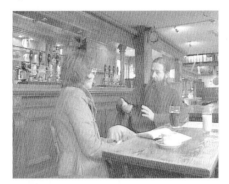

INTERVIEW WITH AUBREY DE GREY

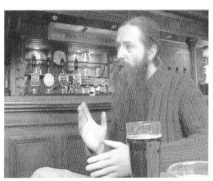

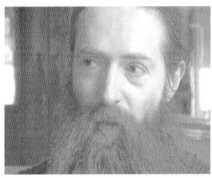

AUBREY

'I take the social context of life extension very seriously. It's clear that if we were to make the sort of breakthroughs that I think we're going to be able to make, then more or less everything about life would be different.'

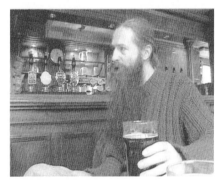

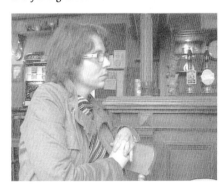

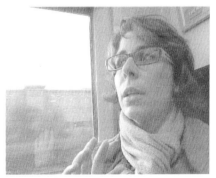

SUSANA

'I don't need to believe his arguments, but there is a certain perception that we are making technologies for a better life, and it's something we have to think about – the implications and the consequences of that.'

3.4.1 *Film stills from Aubrey de Grey interview*

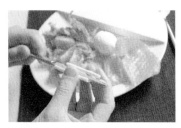

Fig. 3.4.2

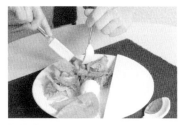

Fig. 3.4.3

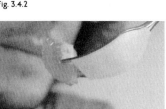

Fig. 3.4.4

WE LIVE

WHAT WE EAT

—

THE SAGB

TABLEWARE

SET

Cutting calories may have an effect on animals' longevity. Recent controversial studies indicated similar results in humans.

The SAGB Tableware Set is complemented with restrictive utensils that can help to reduce the amount of food intake. These were inspired by the adjustable gastric band implants (SAGB) designed for obese patients whose life expectancy is decreased. The band creates a small pouch at the top of the stomach that quickly fills with food. A message is sent to the brain and the person feels full, so eating more slowly, and eating less.

Like the gastric band, the SAGB Tableware Set restricts the amount of food intake, and therefore the person eats more slowly and feels hungry less often.

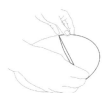

Fig. 3.4.5

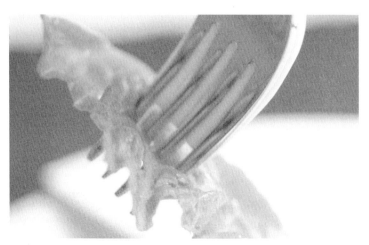

3.4.2–3.4.6 *SAGB tableware designs and scenario*

Fig. 3.4.6

THE VEGETARIAN TOOTH

Teeth are an essential tool for nutrition; their shape is related to diet. The form of herbivore teeth is suited to the grinding of plant material.

It is estimated that meat production accounts for nearly a fifth of greenhouse gas emissions. Recently the UN appealed for a radical shift in diet, to provide individual health benefits and to place less pressure on our global ecology.

Can our tooth structure be modified, to reflect and enhance our dietary preferences?

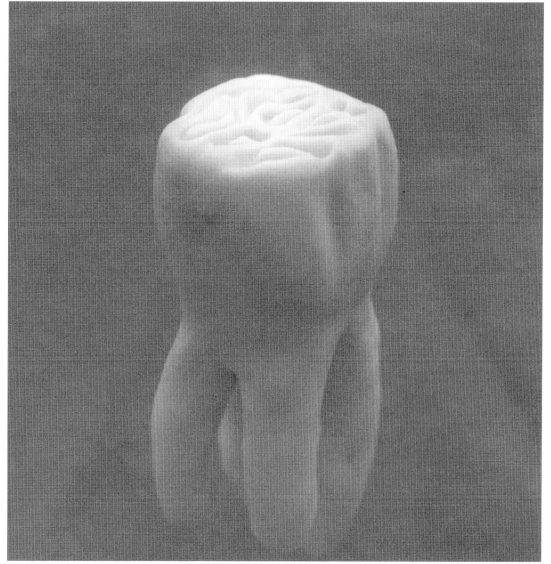

Fig. 3.4.7

3.4.7 *Vegetarian Tooth prototype*

TRANSPLANTATION OF STEM CELLS

'Cells for sight' research is aiming to understand the biology and therapeutic potential of adult stem cells in order to develop and deliver new therapies to patients suffering from blinding ocular surface disorders.

Limbal epithelial cells are harvested through a biopsy of the patient's healthy eye cells. The tissue biopsy is then cultured on amniotic membrane and transplanted onto the patient's cornea – a similar technique to the one used to grow skin.

So far, patients at Moorfields Eye Hospital, have experienced an improvement in their clinical condition following cultured limbal epithelial stem cell transplantation.

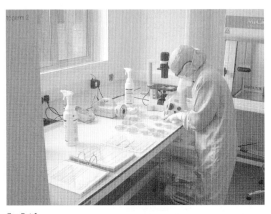

Fig. 3.4.8

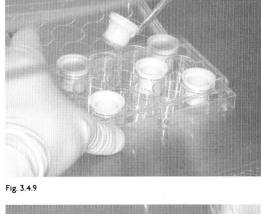

Fig. 3.4.9

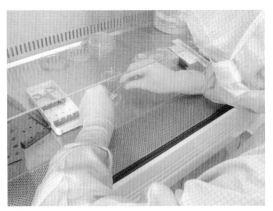

Fig. 3.4.10

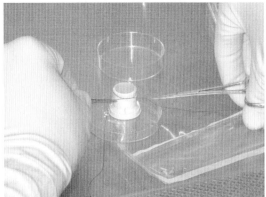

Fig. 3.4.11

3.4.8 *Cleanroom monitoring*
3.4.9 *Place graft in new well to remove media*
3.4.10 *Removing amnion from backing paper*
3.1.11 *Suture*

MATERIAL BELIEFS
INTERACTION RESEARCH STUDIO

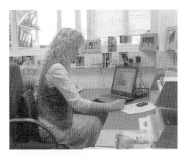

INTERVIEW AT THE INSTITUTE OF OPTHAMOLOGY

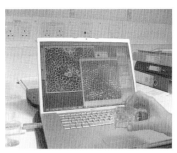

Fig. 3.4.12

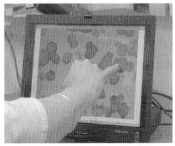

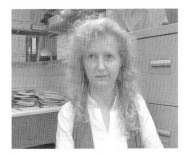

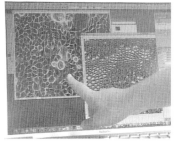

JULIE

Clinically how we are trying to help these patients is by growing their own stem cells in the lab and transplanting them onto the front surface of the eye. This involves taking a small biopsy from the healthy eye... We isolate the cells through a series of enzyme digestions, and we grow those cells up on a substrate, which will then allow us to give those back to the surgeon.

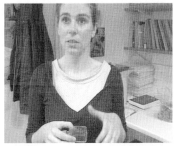

SUSANA

Stem cells research is replacing flesh with flesh, so you replace your deficient cells with your healthy cells. All this could be like your life insurance later on. So that's going to be the second part of the project – what was considered disposable can be reusable and precious now.

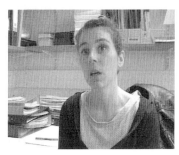

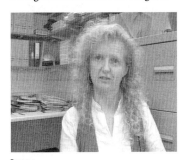

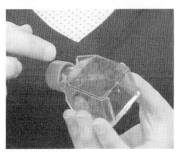

SUSANA

This is like a dead culture of the stem cells. I'm trying to translate these into a 3D structure, so I take pictures of these stem cells and tissue, I put these in the computer and programme, and the computer creates a mesh out of these cells – it's like a translation.

JULIE

This process takes 3-4 weeks. After the patient has had their surgery, they can hopefully see some improvement in their vision after a few weeks.

3.4.12 *Film stills from Bonsai Cells description*

These experimental cell cultures were developed by designer Susana Soares in collaboration with Anna Harris, a PhD student at the Institute of Ophthalmology who is optimising methods of cell culture used in therapies for eye diseases. Julie Daniels, a professor at the Institute, acted as a project advisor.

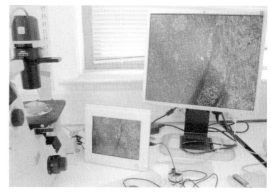

Fig. 3.4.13

BONSAI CELLS

—

DESIGNING CULTURES

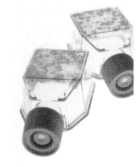

Fig. 3.4.14

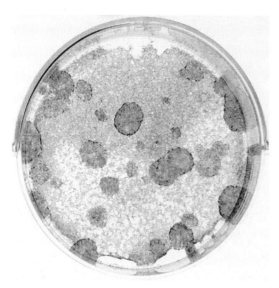

Fig. 3.4.15

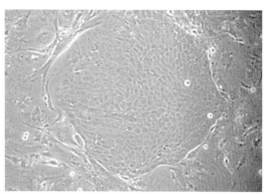

Fig. 3.4.16

Cultured stem cells have contributed to therapeutic treatments. Healthy cells harvested from the patient can be cultured and then transplanted onto failed and abnormal tissue, regenerating the tissue and restoring function. The efficiency of this regeneration is affected by the properties of these cells, how fast they grow, their shape, size and distribution.

3.4.15 *Colonies of stained epithelial stem cells (dead culture)*
3.4.16 *An epithelial stem cell colony surrounded by feeder cells (living culture)*

During culture, the cells can be transformed in a number of ways. They can be reprogrammed to become different types of cells, for example heart muscle cells. The shape of the growing culture can also be influenced – it can be pruned or branched in a manner that recalls the cultivation of bonsai plants.

For these Bonsai cells studies, patterns were designed in 3D software and fabricated as textured surfaces. Colonies of stem cells were then seeded on to four different surfaces and cultured for ten days, then stained with a marker to show how the patterns had affected the culture.

This aesthetic exploration of cell cultures also provides opportunities for medical research, including novel approaches to labelling, marking, measuring and controlling the shape of cell cultures.

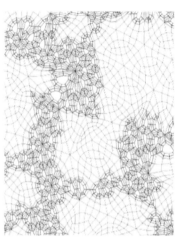

Fig. 3.4.17

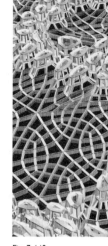

Fig. 3.4.18

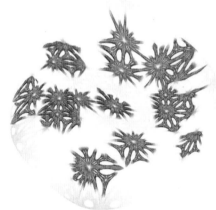

Fig. 3.4.19

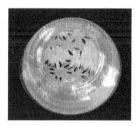

Fig. 3.4.20

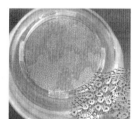

Fig. 3.4.21

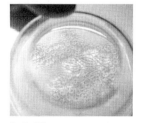

Fig. 3.4.22

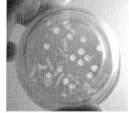

Fig. 3.4.23

3.4.17 *Cultured cell structure study 1*
3.4.18 *Cultured cell structure study 2*
3.4.19 *Stem cell shape study*
3.4.20 *Study for stem epithelial cells structure*
3.4.21 *Study for stem skin cells structure 1*
3.4.22 *Study for stem skin cells structure 2*
3.4.23 *Study for stem eye cell structure*

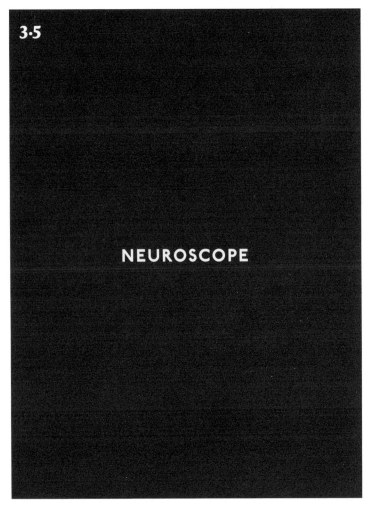

3·5

NEUROSCOPE

This project was a collaboration between Victor Becerra, Julia Downes, Mark Hammond, Slawomir Jaroslaw Nasuto, Kevin Warwick, Ben Whalley and Dimitris Xydas – researchers and doctoral students schools of Pharmacy and Systems Engineering at Reading University – and designers Elio Caccavale and David Muth.

The Neuroscope situates features pharmacy and cybernetics research in a domestic product, thus provoking questions about the possibility of linking objects in the home to material in the lab.

Neuroscope exemplifies one possible future relationship with an emergent class of living assemblages – entities that are classed as neither organism nor object.

'I remember going away from one of these meetings with this big headache – how on earth am I going to make everybody happy?'

ELIO CACCAVALE
Interaction Research Studio, Goldsmiths

'You can be provocative, but you've got to be provocative within the letter of the law.'

BEN WHALLERY
School of Pharmacy, University of Reading

ANIMAT

—

CONTROLLING A ROBOT WITH NEURONES

Fig. 3.5.1

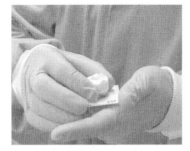

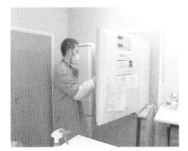

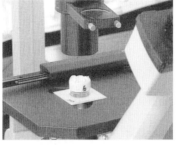

DIMITRIUS
On one side you'd have robots with actually biological brains, and on the other side you'd hopefully have medical applications.

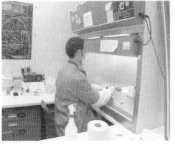

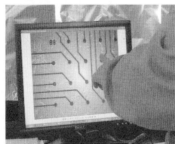

MARK
The project is to understand network level processing in a neurone network. We want to understand how they interact to process signals, basically.

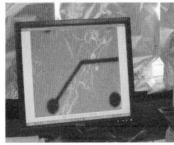

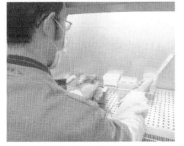

3.5.1 *Film stills from Neuroscope meeting at University of Reading*

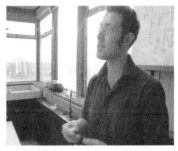

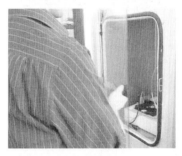

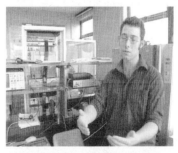

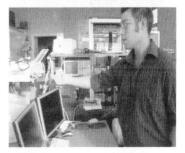

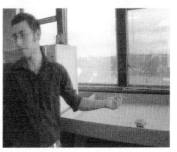

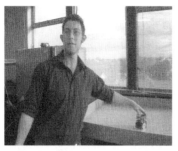

MARK
The idea is that the culture is in charge of its own behaviour. It is able to interact with the environment and the consequences of its decision affect future decisions. This is the robot moving around under control of the culture, so when you see it make another change in direction, that's because something has changed in the culture, so at one electrode cells are firing at a slightly higher frequency, which makes it go to the right, for example.

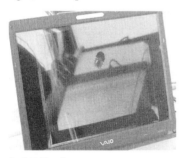

Fig. 3.5.1 (Cont.)

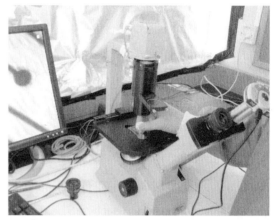

Fig. 3.5.2

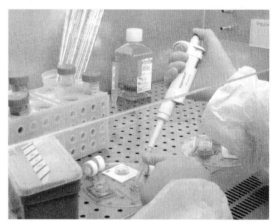

Fig. 3.5.3

3.5.2 – 3.5.4 *Cells settle on the bottom of the Multi Electrode Array (MEA) and form connections. Electrodes embedded in to the substrate allow recording of the electrical signals produced by the cells*

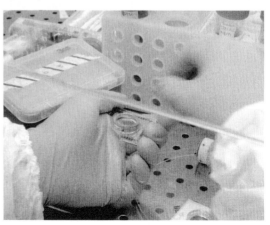

Fig. 3.5.4

MATERIAL BELIEFS
INTERACTION RESEARCH STUDIO

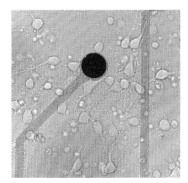

Fig. 3.5.5

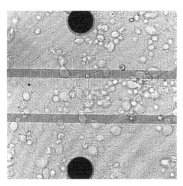

Fig. 3.5.6

3.5.5 – 3.5.6 *Cells (irregular shapes) grow on an MEA dish with a carpet of connections between them. Recording of electrical activity is undertaken through the electrodes (large black circle)*
3.5.7 – 3.5.8 *The robot acts as the body. It is equipped with sonar and light sensors which act as the culture's sensory input whilst the culture's output controls the wheel speed and direction*
3.5.9 *These vertical waveforms show the electrical activity of the cells, where large changes could be used to trigger signals to be sent to the robot*

Fig. 3.5.7

Fig. 3.5.8

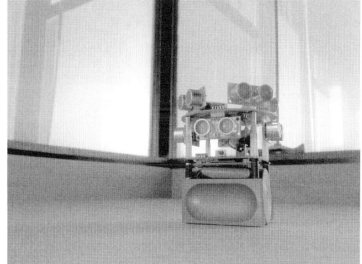

Fig. 3.5.9

Fig. 3.5.10

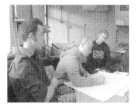

DISCUSSION AT THE UNIVERSITY OF READING

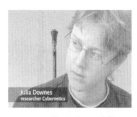

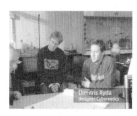

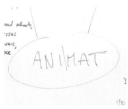

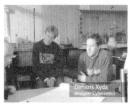

ELIO
Why is it called Animat? Because I think it has been used by other people as well.

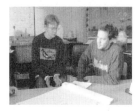

MARK
Animat is a concept in AI that means creating an artificial body.

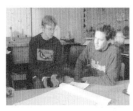

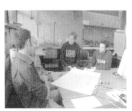

JULIA
You could define whether it works in a number of ways. It could work in the way that we are getting to understand how the cultures are working much better, or we create a really good robot controller that redefines the way that people program robots.

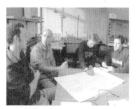

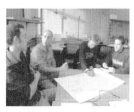

DIMITRIUS
The more you learn about the underlying neurons themselves, the more you can use that in applications.

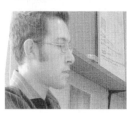

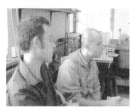

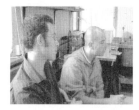

ELIO
How would you see this used? In what kind of format?

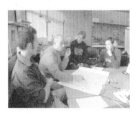

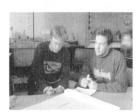

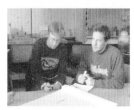

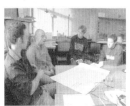

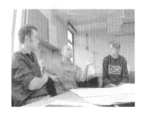

3.5.10 *Film stills from Neuroscope meeting at University of Reading*

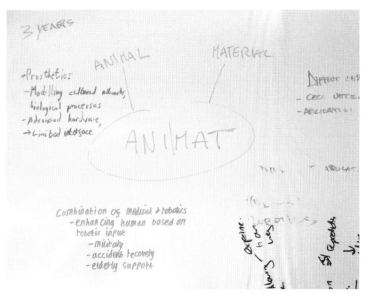

Fig. 3.5.11

3.5.11 – 3.5.12 *Drawings made during the discussion detailing alternative uses for interfaces between cells and objects.*

SKETCHES

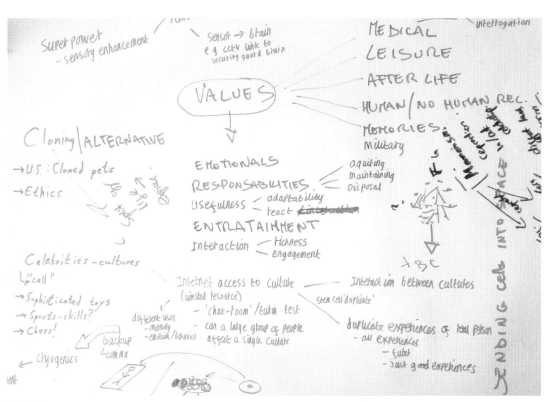

Fig. 3.5.12

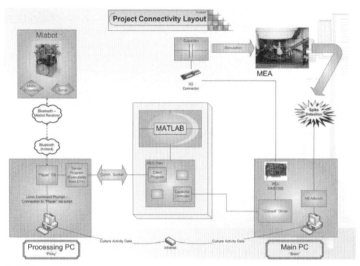

3.5.13 *Diagram for an academic paper – a system linking a culture of cells to a robot*
3.5.14 *Reinterpreting the system to link the cells in a lab to a product in the home*
3.5.15 *Research leaves the lab in the form of products – some are imminent and plausible, others more distant and fantastic*

Fig. 3.5.13

SYSTEMS

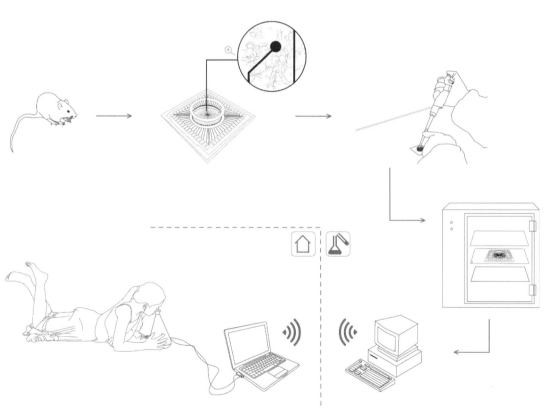

Fig. 3.5.14

MATERIAL BELIEFS
INTERACTION RESEARCH STUDIO

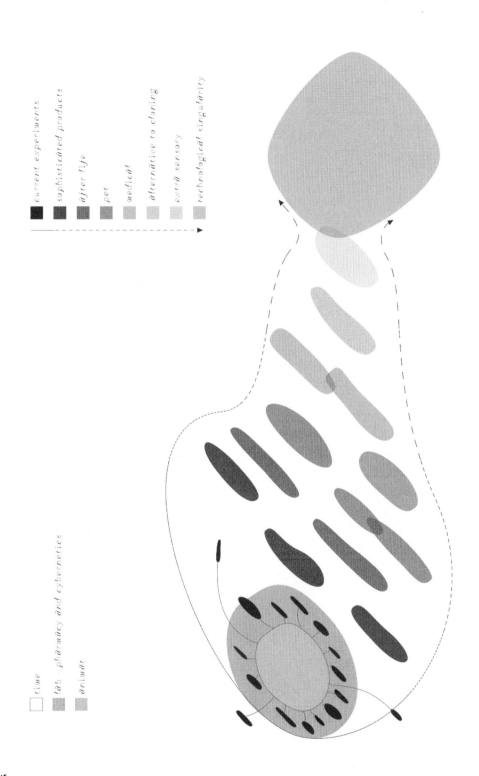

Fig. 3.5.15

3.5.16 – 3.5.19 *Testing the form of the Neuroscope with card and paper*

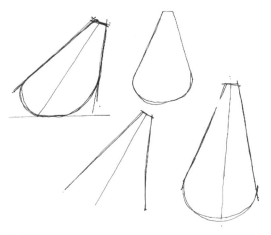

Fig. 3.5.16

CARD

MODELS

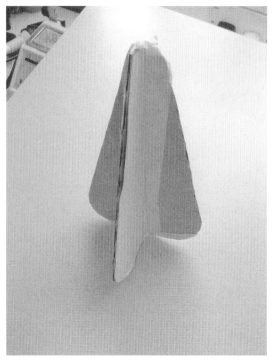

Fig. 3.5.17

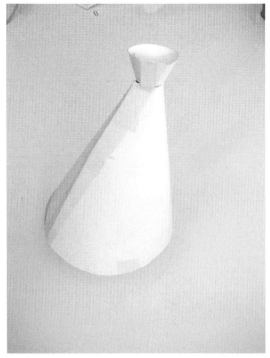

Fig. 3.5.18

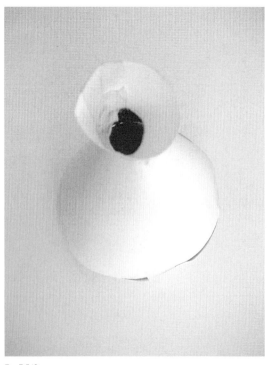

Fig. 3.5.19

MATERIAL BELIEFS
INTERACTION RESEARCH STUDIO

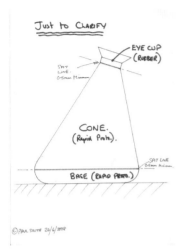

Fig. 3.5.20

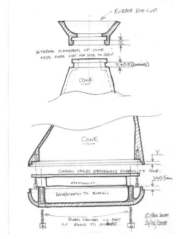

Fig. 3.5.21

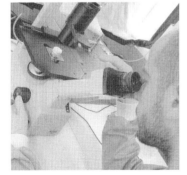

Fig. 3.5.22

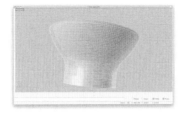

Fig. 3.5.23

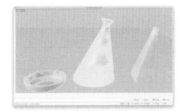

Fig. 3.5.24

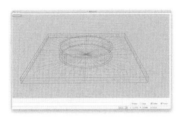

Fig. 3.5.25

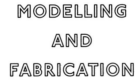

MODELLING
AND
FABRICATION

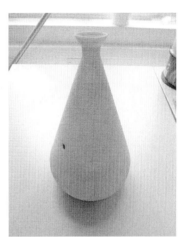

Fig. 3.5.26

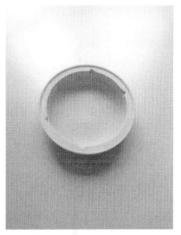

Fig. 3.5.27

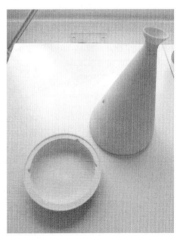

Fig. 3.5.28

3.5.20 – 3.5.21 *Diagrams of the prototype from the model maker*
3.5.22 *Laboratory imaging tools informed the design*
3.5.23 – 3.5.25 *Modelling the body in CAD software*
3.5.26 – 3.5.28 *Finished Neuroscope body*

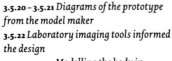

NEUROSCOPE
DESCRIPTION

'The aim was to develop an interface that
had a meaningful relationship with the
behaviour of the cell culture.'
ELIO CACCAVALE
Interaction Research Studio, Goldsmiths

Fig. 3.5.29

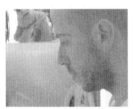
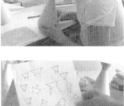
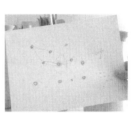
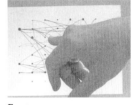

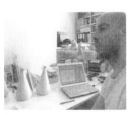
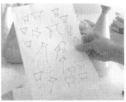
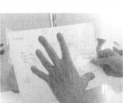

ELIO
As you interact with it you
will be sending signals
to the cell culture, which
then will feedback into the
virtual environment, so
there is a loop between what
you do with the Neuroscope
and the cell culture.

ELIO
The idea was to develop
some sort of interactive
device to interact with
the cell culture from the
home, by using the form of
a microscope, something
which is familiar in a
lab environment, and
bringing that language
and transforming it to a
domestic environment

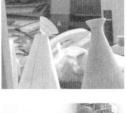
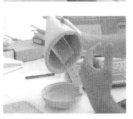
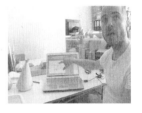

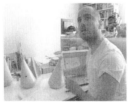

ELIO
What we came up with
was something called the
Neuroscope. When you look
into it you will be able to see
this virtual representation,
which is updating in real
time, because the object
is networked to the cell
culture in the lab.

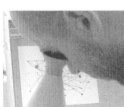
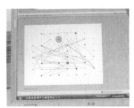
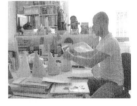

Fig. 3.5.29 *Film stills from Neuroscope
description*

MATERIAL BELIEFS
INTERACTION RESEARCH STUDIO

SOFTWARE
SKETCHES

> '**I have been working on algorithmic visualisations of neural activity. This project is of particular interest to me, as it touches on philosophical questions about consciousness and decision making.**'
> DAVID MUTH
> *Design Interactions, Royal College of Art*

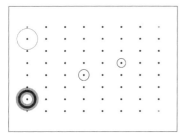

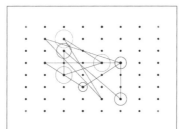

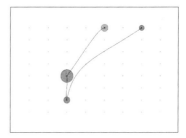

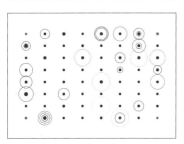

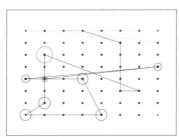

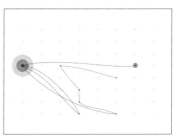

Stage 01.01

An 8x8 grid of electrodes detecting neural activity in a culture of brain tissue.
Fig. 3.5.30 and Fig. 3.5.31

Stage 01.03

In an initial meeting with the scientific team, Mark Hammond remarked that consecutive bursts at given locations could be interpreted as an indicator for existing neural connection between those locations. Fig. 3.5.32 and Fig. 3.5.33

Stage 01.06

Fig. 3.5.34 and Fig. 3.5.35

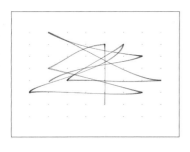

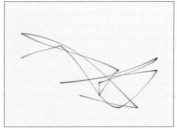

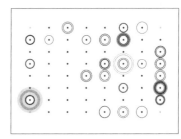

Stage 01.17

A more tissue-like look after feedback on previous sketches from Mark Hammond.
Fig. 3.5.36

Stage 01.24

Fig. 3.5.37

Stage 02.06

Refinement of initial versions of the visualisation, after further feedback from the scientific team. Fig. 3.5.38

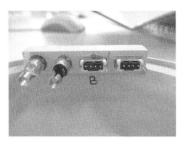

Fig. 3.5.39

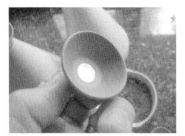

Fig. 3.5.40

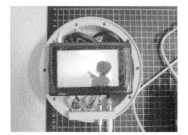

Fig. 3.5.41

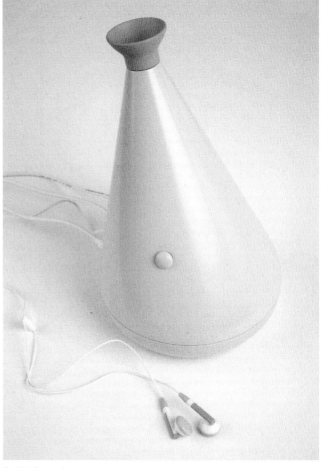

Fig. 3.5.42

NEUROSCOPE
PROTOTYPE

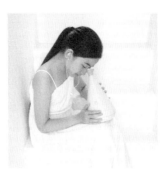

Fig. 3.5.43

3.5.39 – 3.5.41 *Fitting connectors*
and electronics
3.5.42 *Final prototype*
3.5.43 – 3.5.44 *Using the Neuroscope*
at home

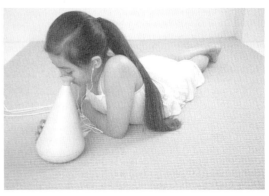

Fig. 3.5.44

MATERIAL BELIEFS
INTERACTION RESEARCH STUDIO

Chapter 4

THE CREDIBLE
AND
THE INCREDIBLE

—

PROVOKING

DEBATE

4.0

THE CREDIBLE
AND
THE INCREDIBLE
—
PROVOKING
DEBATE

'For me, it has mostly been about changing – changing the boundaries that we use to describe things … Stop thinking about what's credible and think about what might be incredible. Hey, how's that for a sound bite? You can use it if you like.'
NICK OLIVER
Institute of Biomedical Engineering, Imperial College London

'You can't ask questions at an exhibition unless there's somebody there to ask.'
JULIE DANIELS
Institute of Ophthalmology

Surprising people is one thing, provoking debate another. In order to have a debate, you need to have people who are ready and willing to talk to each other. With this in mind, we tried to *design* our second round of public engagements. Our aim was, within the constraints of each event, to optimise discussion. The more, the merrier. And the more diverse the participants, the greater the chances of unexpected insights. Better yet, hand out felt-tips and plasticine …

This chapter documents those public engagements and people's responses, and then presents an essay reflecting on the social dynamics of the collaborative process in Material Beliefs, as evinced by focus groups held in December 2008. One can also reflect on the individual experiences of those involved, with an eye to the future. What will result from people's experiences of the project? How does this differ for participants and spectators, or are spectators also participants? In other words, what do we – or they – *do* with these experiences? Can we ever say for sure? And even if we could, how do we measure the success of the project as a whole?

Such subjective questions are difficult to approach, and certainly can't be framed in the terms which Emily Dawson uses in her essay – and this raises a final, key question about Material Beliefs. To put it bluntly, is 'critical design' here paying lip service to sociological models of 'public engagement of science'? Is it, essentially, presenting art in the guise of science? Or is something else going on, as Mike Michael suggests in the opening essay: 'what emerges is not "solutions" but better problems'?

The book ends with appendices: events, dates, names.

So many names. These pages are scattered with names, of engineers and designers and academics and volunteers and audience members … As we said in the first chapter, there are many interesting, and potentially interested, people out there. If you're reading this book, you're one of them. Perhaps you'd never heard of Material Beliefs before picking up the book. If so, what do *you* do with the experience?

4.1

LATER PUBLIC ENGAGEMENT EVENTS

The project again moved out into public arenas, this time with the designs. The prototypes were the subject of a second evening event at the Dana Centre, an exhibition at a festival in Zagreb, and a Channel 4 News broadcast at the Kinetica Art Fair.

'One of our problems with this critical design area is that it remains very much within a design realm. Our goal ought to be to disseminate our work to as broad a public as possible, so you can get a true response from the people whom these technologies and their applications are going to impact.'

JIMMY LOIZEAU
Department of Design, Goldsmiths

EMILY: And what do you want to get out of doing public engagement?
MARK: Publicity for research. The opportunity to potentially – if we do it correctly – gain insights from the public or experts who may turn up, that we wouldn't otherwise get – and the light bulb wouldn't have gone on if we'd just been sitting round the table having our usual conversations.

MARK HAMMOND   AND   EMILY DAWSON
Department of Mechanical Engineering,   *Department of Education and Professional*
University College London   *Studies, King's College London*

BIO PLAY AT DANA

4.1.1 – 4.1.3 *Discussing cells as aesthetic materials*
4.1.4 *Dana Centre press release*

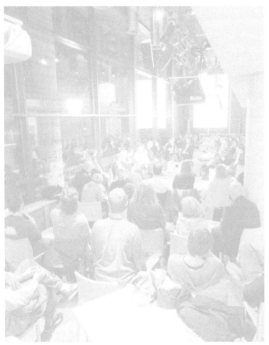

Fig. 4.1.1

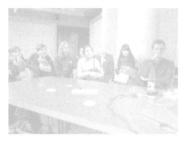

Fig. 4.1.2

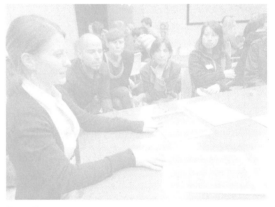

Fig. 4.1.3

BIO PLAY
28 October 2008

How can playfulness expand horizons in bioengineering? What happens when we open up laboratories to the whim of undefined ends, exploration and wonder? What are the benefits and dangers of designers engaging with medical science? By expanding current laboratory research through speculative designs, Material Beliefs aim to create prototypes that redraw the intersection between science, engineering and design and lead to new realms of thought. Discuss these intriguing projects and question the novel collaborations that conceived them.

Event organised by the Science Museum

'I don't think exhibitions are very engaging, and in the future I want to challenge that method because what I thought worked better – and we only had one chance to do it – was at the Dana Centre.'
SUSANA SOARES
Interaction Research Studio, Goldsmiths

'You end up with a very self-selecting, smallish group of public who go to all these events, and they're all very interested and very bright and very knowledgeable and very erudite, but is that really public engagement?'
NICK OLIVER
Institute of Biomedical Engineering, Imperial College London

Fig. 4.1.4

TOUCH ME! FESTIVAL – FEEL BETTER!
19–23 December 2008

The Touch Me project is concerned with art at the intersection of science and technology. It was formed by the group KONTEJNER in 2002, became a festival in 2005, and this year's festival has a name with connotations of pleasure – *Feel Better!*

The festival explores how the individual can be bound into the network of electronics, cybernetics and biotechnology, and how these networks become challenged by the individual's need for happiness, pleasure and hedonism.

Fig. 4.1.5

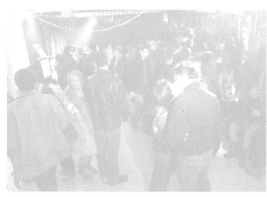

Fig. 4.1.6

TOUCH ME!
EXHIBITION

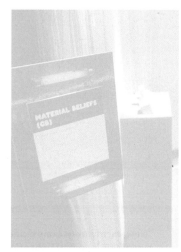

Fig. 4.1.7

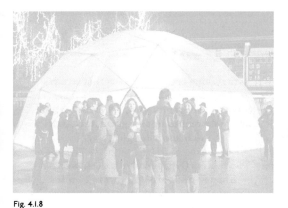

Fig. 4.1.8

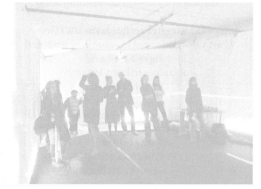

4.1.5 – 4.1.9 *Live performance and presentations accompanied the exhibition*

Fig. 4.1.9

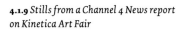
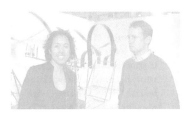

4.1.9 *Stills from a Channel 4 News report on Kinetica Art Fair*

CDER
CHANNEL 4
NEWS

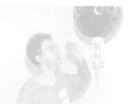

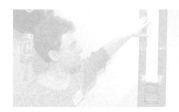

Fig. 4.1.9

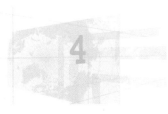
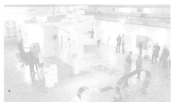
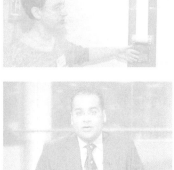

'Now, carnivorous lampshades, sculptures made from beams of light and pole-dancing robots – just some of the curiosities on display at an exhibition opening today.'

'The Kinetica art fair is the UK's first art show dedicated to robotic, sound- and light-based art.'
KRISHNAN GURU-MURTHY
Channel 4 News

'The artists here reference the past as well as incorporating new technology from the future.'
TONY LANGFORD
Kinetica Art Fair

'So this is a lampshade robot that attracts insects inside by the light that's there already. They get trapped, fall to the bottom, and by decomposing they generate electricity that keep the light going.'

'So this is a flypaper robotic clock, we have a honey-covered band, once in a while a motor rotates, any insects that are caught in it are scraped off into the fuel cell at the bottom, where it generates electricity for a clock, and we can watch the flies approaching their inevitable death in the fuel cell, for entertainment value.'
ALEKSANDAR ZIVANOVIC
Freelance design engineer

4.2

ROYAL INSTITUTION EXHIBITION AND FAMILY DAY

Crossing Over was an exhibition staged throughout the newly refurbished Royal Institution of Great Britain building.

Material Beliefs joined Anne Brodie, Alex Bunn, Eggebert-and-Gould, Kathleen Rogers, Carl Stevenson and Phoebe von Held as exhibitors. The show explored exchanges in art and biotechnology, and was curated by Caterina Albano and Rowan Drury of Artakt, Central Saint Martins College of Art and Design.

During the exhibition, collaborators also took part in an evening of debate about the culture of art and science, and set up a studio during 'Family Fun Day', where young visitors designed their own biological robots.

'Jimmy, James and Alex have their carnivorous domestic entertainment robots installed at the Royal Institution. It's a Saturday, it's family day. We've designed an activity around these fly-eating robots. What we're asking the children to do is design their own robots, and the questions we're asking them are: how do they catch the fly, where is the stomach, and then once the robot's eaten the fly what's the electricity for?'

TOBIE KERRIDGE
Department of Design, Goldsmiths

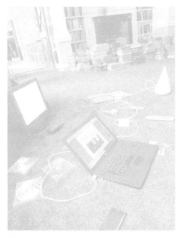

Fig. 4.2.1

THE
EXHIBITION

'In commenting on the flourishing of bio-art, Dominique Lestel observes, "Some of the most creative artistic practices today are resolutely engaged in the manipulation of life forms. It is a fascinating tendency. A disturbing one too."'

'The same could be said of "biodesign", as an innovative field where cutting-edge scientific and technological experimentation meets speculative design. The result is an intriguing, possibly perplexing projection of the potential applications of biotechnological developments. Similar to bio-art, biodesign also results from collaborations and takes biotechnological material outside the laboratory into the public domain – through art galleries and beyond. Still removed from the dynamics of mass production, biodesign presents prototypes for intellectual rather than utilitarian consumption.'

'Yet, the language and approach are distinctively those of design in the synthesis of material, object and social systems. At the interface of science and social technologies, of application and communication, biodesign uses bio-artifacts to explore the integration of biomaterials within everyday environments, encouraging new modes of engagement with the changing spectrum of life forms. Within the context of *Crossing Over*, Material Beliefs represent this emergent field of collaborative design practice.'

CATERINA ALBANO
Extract from exhibition catalogue

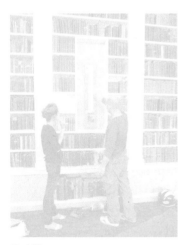

Fig. 4.2.2

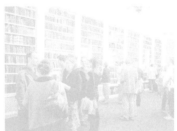

Fig. 4.2.3

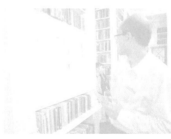

Fig. 4.2.4

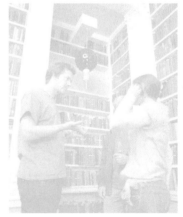

Fig. 4.2.5

4.2.1 – 4.2.2 *Installing work at the Royal Institution*
4.2.3 – 4.2.5 *Exhibition opening*
4.2.6 – 4.2.10 *Robots designed by children at Family Fun Day*

FLY-EATING ROBOTS AT FAMILY FUN DAY

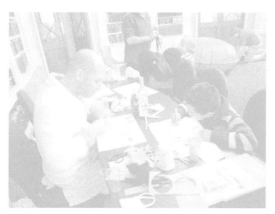

Fig. 4.2.6

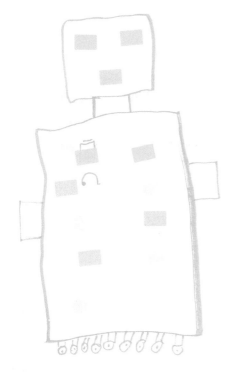

Fig. 4.2.8

NOVEMBER 08 FAMILY FUN DAY

Saturday 1 November 2008
Drop in between 11.00a.m. and 4.00p.m.
Suitable for 5-14 year olds

The November Family Fun Day is themed around Halloween, and we have a fancy dress competition running. Come and scare us as a witch, ghost or mad scientist!

Our new Family Fun Days continue, where the whole family can immerse themselves in science! Drop in between 11.00a.m. and 4.00p.m. on the first Saturday of every month to see, hear, smell and touch science with a range of hands-on activities, exciting demonstrations and captivating talks. From eggsperiments and DNA to the world's largest whoopee cushion there is something to keep the whole family entertained. You can even join Michael Faraday on an interactive tour of our new exhibition to seek out the treasures of the Ri. After all that you will probably have worked up quite an appetite, so why not grab some lunch or a tasty bite in our brand new café?

Fig. 4.2.7

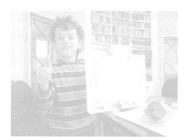

Fig. 4.2.9

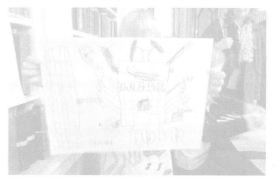

Fig. 4.2.10

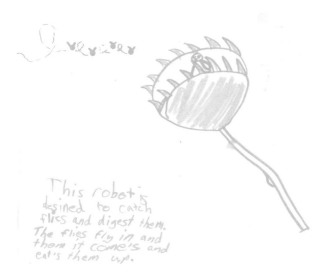

This robot is designed to catch flies and digest them. The flies fly in and them it come's and eat's them up.

Fig. 4.2.11

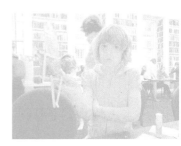

Fig. 4.2.12

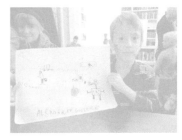

Fig. 4.2.13

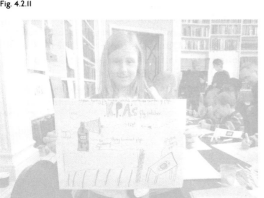

Fig. 4.2.14

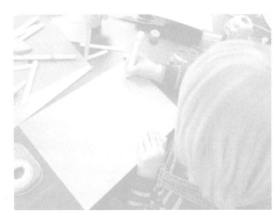

Fig. 4.2.15

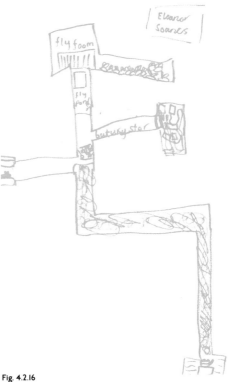

Fig. 4.2.16

Fig. 4.2.17

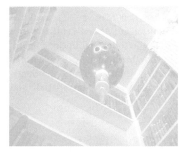
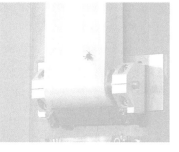
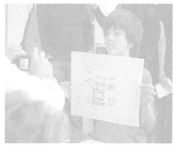

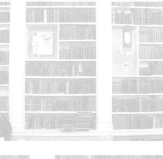
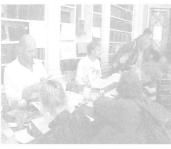
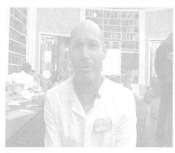

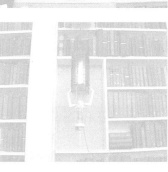
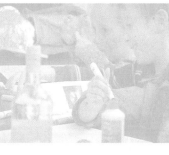
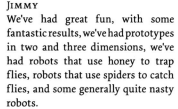

Jimmy
We've had great fun, with some fantastic results, we've had prototypes in two and three dimensions, we've had robots that use honey to trap flies, robots that use spiders to catch flies, and some generally quite nasty robots.

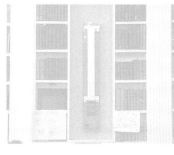
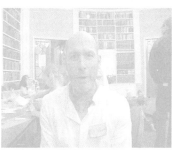
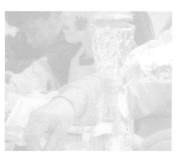

4.2.11 – 4.2.16 *Robots designed by children at Family Fun Day*
4.2.17 *Film stills from Family day at the Royal Institution*

4·3

NOWHERE/NOW/HERE

—

EXHIBITION

AT LABORAL

Designs from the Material Beliefs collaborations were featured in *Nowhere/Now/Here*, an international exhibition at LABoral Centro de Arte y Creación Industrial in Gijon Spain. The show featured more than 60 works ranging from everyday products, fashion, jewellery to installations and live performances.

'Our intent was to present a collection of objects that would allow you to understand the thinking process of the artists behind them. Presenting them as thinkers who can not only reshape their own particular worlds but show the potential to transform, reinterpret and rethink industries, production processes, communication strategies, political systems, etc Challenging our preconceptions of what design can do.'

ROBERTO FEO   AND   ROSARIO HURTADO
Curator, Nowhere/Now/Here   *Curator, Nowhere/Now/Here*

'I always struggle to find the purpose of an exhibition. Is it for the sake of having to tick a box – I had a show, it's good for my CV? And quite often what works well is the opening: you are there and you can engage with all sorts of people. You might have mums and dads coming because they're interested, but you might also have an expert who hasn't been involved with that kind of work, or isn't familiar with art and design. But then, you know what happens afterwards: other visitors come but you're not there to explain the work.'

ELIO CACCAVALE
Interaction Research Studio, Goldsmiths

Fig. 4.3.1 *Nowhere/Now/Here invitation (page 1)*

LABoral Centro de Arte y Creación Industrial

se complace en invitarle a la Inauguración de:
is pleased to invite you to the Opening of:

NOWHERE/NOW/HERE
09.10.2008 – 20.04.2009

Explorando nuevas líneas de investigación en el diseño contemporáneo
Investigating new lines of enquiry in contemporary design

Una exposición comisariada por:
An exhibition curated by:
Roberto Feo & Rosario Hurtado
(El Último Grito)

Artistas: *Artists:*
5:5 Designers, AA, Amidov, Assa
Ashuach, Bruce Bell, Bryony Birkbeck,
Tord Boontje, Marta Botas & Germán R.
Blanco, David Bowen, Fernando Brizio,
Nacho Carbonell, Daniel Charny &
Gabriel Klasmer, Santiago Cirugeda, Carl
Clerkin, Paul Cocksedge, Dainippon Type
Organization, Óscar Díaz, Dunne & Raby,
Daniel Eatock, Olivia Flore Decaris, Tiago
Fonseca, Fulguro & Thomas Jomini

Architecture Workshop, Martino Gamper,
Martí Guixé, Mathias Hahn, Interaction
Research Studio, Onkar Kular,
Tithi Kutchamuch, Dash MacDonald,
Material Beliefs (Auger-Loizeau, Elio
Caccavale, Tobie Kerridge, David Muth,
Susana Soares, Aleksandar Zivanovic),
Alejandro Mazuelas, Alon Meron,
mmmm..., Eelko Moorer, Oscar Narud,
NB: Studio, Ernesto Oroza, Marc Owens,
Pedrita, Laura Potter, Corinne Quin,
Random International, Raw Edges Design
Studio, Nic Rysenbry, Jerszy Seymour,
Bert Simons, Studio Glithero, Yuri Suzuki,
Gregor Timlin, Noam Toran, Manel
Torres, Maud Traon, Troika, Pablo

Valbuena, Greetje van Helmond,
Dominic Wilcox, Nick Williamson,
Marei Wollersberger, Zaunka

Agradecimientos especiales a:
Special thanks to:
Ron Arad, Javier Mariscal,
Gaetano Pesce, Daniel Weil

Diseño de la exposición:
Exhibition design:
Patricia Urquiola & Martino Berghinz

Diseño gráfico: *Graphic design:*
Fernando Gutiérrez

Que tendrá lugar el 9 de octubre de 2008, a las 20 horas
Taking place on 9th October 2008, at 8 pm

LABoral Centro de Arte y Creación Industrial
Los Prados, 121
33394 Gijón
Asturias
T. +34 985 185 577
F. +34 985 337 355
info@laboralcentrodearte.org
www.laboralcentrodearte.org

Horario del Centro: miércoles a lunes, de 12 a 20 horas
Opening Hours: Wednesday to Monday, from 12 noon to 8 pm

Invitación válida para dos personas. Se ruega presentación a la entrada
Valid for 2. Please bring this invitation with you

Centro de Arte y Creación Industrial

Fig. 4.3.2 *Nowhere/Now/Here invitation (page 2)*

4.2.3 *Nowhere/Now/Here
exhibition lobby*
4.2.4 *Neuroscope at Nowhere/
Now/Here*
4.2.5 *Lampshade Robot at
Nowhere/Now/Here*

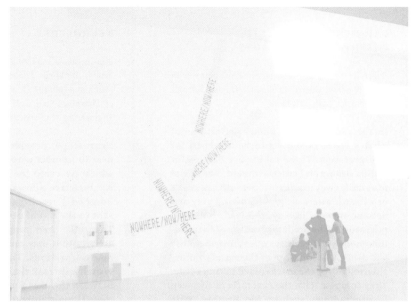

Fig. 4.3.3

THE
EXHIBITION

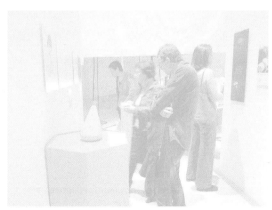

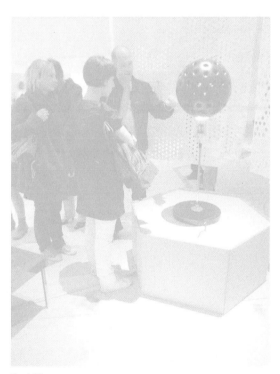

Fig. 4.3.4

Fig. 4.3.5

CARNIVOROUS DOMESTIC ENTERTAINMENT ROBOTS

Auger-Loizeau and Aleksandar Zivanovic, with Julian Vincent, Centre for Biomimetic and Natural Technologies, Bath University

In the context of the home, definitions of what a robot is and could be are open for interpretation. These robots are devices for utility, drama and entertainment. They exist in a similar way to an exotic pet such as a snake or a lizard, where we provide living prey and become voyeurs in a synthesized, contrived microcosm. The predatory nature of these autonomous entities raises questions about life and death, taking us out of the moral comfort zone regarding the mechanised taking of life. They compete with the spectacle of life seen in programmes such as Big Brother, Wife Swap or televised, edited and dramatised depictions of war. As consumers of these programmes, like those who keep vivariums, we have the potential to be repulsed, engaged or both, and as voyeurs might consider ourselves complicit.

Fig. 4.3.6

NEUROSCOPE

Elio Caccavale and David Muth, with Kevin Warwick, Ben J. Whalley, Slawomir J. Nasuto, Mark W. Hammond, Julia H. Downes, Dimitris Xydas, School of Pharmacy and Cybernetics, School of Systems Engineering, University of Reading

Neuroscope provides an interface for a user to interact with a culture of brain cells which are cared for in a distant laboratory. An interface allows the virtual cells to be 'touched', resulting in electrical signals sent to the actual neurons in the laboratory. The cells then respond with changes in activity that may result in the formation of new connections. The user experiences this visually in real time, enabling interaction between the user and cell culture as part of a closed loop of interaction.

The project proposes a novel relationship between the laboratory and the home, locating complex scientific processes within everyday life. In this context, a new generation of interactive devices such as Neuroscope emerge, which blur the boundaries between consumer products and biological systems.

Fig. 4.3.7

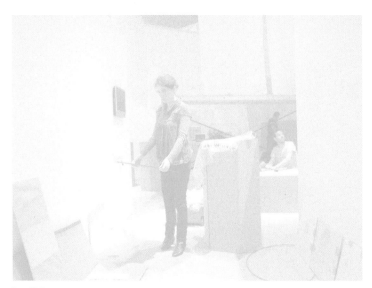

Fig. 4.3.8

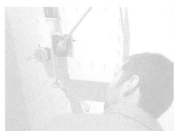

Fig. 4.3.9

4.2.6, 4.3.7, 4.3.10, 4.3.11 *Caption from the installation*
4.2.8 *Unpacking and installing work*
4.2.9 *Checking electronics on the Fly-Stealing Robot*
4.2.12 – 4.3.14 *Exhibition opening*

VITAL SIGNS

Tobie Kerridge, with Tony Cass, Olive Murphy and Nick Oliver, Institute of Biomedical, Imperial College London

The digital plaster incorporates miniature sensors into a skin-worn patch, transmitting data about the body across a mobile phone network. The technology affords new biomedical services, potentially providing live monitoring for patients with chronic conditions, including diabetes and heart conditions.

Vital Signs explores the influence of this technology on the child surveillance industry, where tracking and location services would be extended by incorporating live signals, indicating the temperature, respiration, pulse and orientation of the child's body. Situated within an industry which emphasises risk and provides an opportunity for uninterrupted surveillance, Vital Signs shows how absent bodies are transformed into data and broadcast across networks to become persistently present.

Fig. 4.3.10

WE LIVE WHAT WE EAT

Susana Soares, with Thomas Kirkwood, João Passos, Dianne Ford and Luisa Wakeling, Newcastle University

Studies have demonstrated the benefits of caloric restriction on lifespan. Eating a nutritionally balanced diet, low in calories, is known to slow the biological ageing process in mammals, helping them to live longer and healthier lives. In humans, calorie restriction has been shown to lower cholesterol and blood pressure. Previous successful trials led recently to a study in humans, to better understand the effects of food restriction. Individuals have independently adopted the practice of calorie restriction in some form, hoping to achieve the expected benefits themselves. These approaches have led to debate within the scientific community about public perception and appropriation of scientific research. We Live What We Eat reinterprets these tensions through tableware and palate enhancing utensils to contrive new interactions at mealtimes, which affect our eating habits.

Fig. 4.3.11

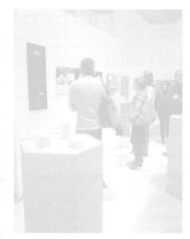

Fig. 4.3.12

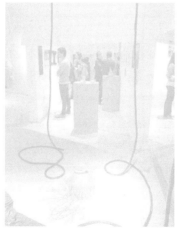

Fig. 4.3.13

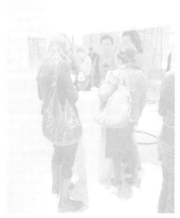

Fig. 4.3.14

4·4

ROUNDHOUSE CYBORG FILM

A Group of young film-makers from the Roundhouse visited the Institute of Biomedical Engineering to film interviews with researchers. A group of three young people and their tutor interviewed Olive Murphy about an implantable blood pressure monitor, Patrick Degenaar about prosthetic vision systems, and Nick Oliver about the development of an artificial pancreas.

'Suddenly they realised, "Oh, these are real researchers. It's not all science fiction from Star Trek." I think that, by the time they were doing the third interview, they had an idea of what was actually going on. It was interesting to see how they adapted, and how they became more sophisticated in their questioning.'

TOBIE KERRIDGE
Interaction Research Studio, Goldsmiths, discusses the experience of engaging with teenagers at an event at the Roundhouse

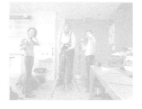
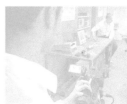
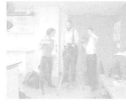
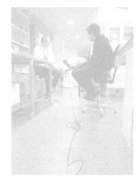

'I work with young people 13-19 years old on a project called TV live. A ten-week course resulting in 4 live TV shows approximately 10 minutes long. The four topics are:

1 Death of Language
2 Heavy Metal
3 Artist Film
4 Cyborgs

Cyborgs and heavy metal are two topics we gave the group to work on, the other two are their own choices.

The course involves pre filming for clips in the live show, to be used in the structure of a show ie. talk show, review show, debate, etc. A good percentage of the group are presently between school and college or university. So they are very are available for a weekday visit to the labs etc.

We are going to do vox pops of views from people on the street about their thoughts reactions to cyberware, and the progression of technology. It would be great to visit labs interview scientist types. Is it possible to get computer visuals of designs etc to insert into programme?

It would be good to hear researchers discuss their sci-fi imaginings, and the reality of technological development.'

OLIVER BANCROFT
Tutor at the Roundhouse, from an email

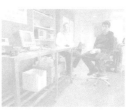
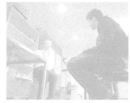
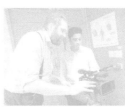
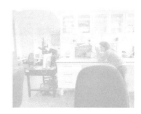
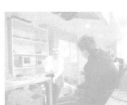
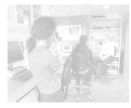
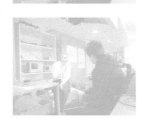
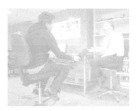
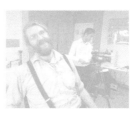

4.4.1 Interviewing researchers at the institute of Biomedical Engineering

Fig. 4.4.1

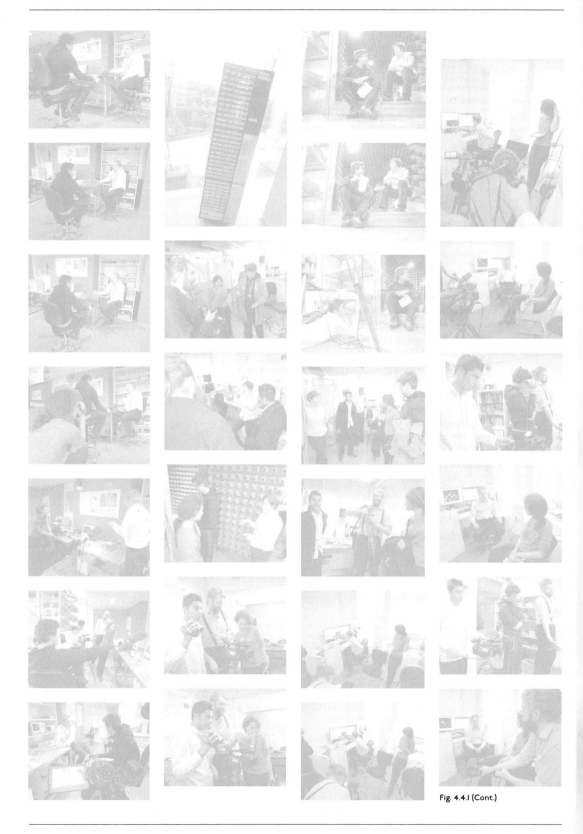

Fig. 4.4.1 (Cont.)

"The idea a few years ago of having a biological silicon hybrid was science fiction, but now because silicon technologies are getting smaller, and our understanding of biological systems is getting better, one can actually see how you can put the two together"

Cyborgs - fact and fiction?
A project with TV Live at the
Roundhouse and the Institute of
Biomedical Engineering, Imperial
College London.

above: quote from Professor Tony
Cass, Deputy Director and Research
Director, Institute of Biomedical
Engineering, Imperial College London,
interviewed June 6th 2007.

Material
Beliefs

EPSRC
Engineering and Physical Sciences
Research Council

Goldsmiths
UNIVERSITY OF LONDON

Fig. 4.4.2 *Information sheet for young people*

Hi Patrick, Olive and Nick

Just a quick catch up about Tuesday 11 November afternoon at IBE. Each interview will only be about 15 minutes, but we'll need to allow some set up time for the equipment. It would also be great to film a quick tour if that is possible?

Here's a provisional plan:
1:30–2:00 Meet, coffee (you're welcome to come along if you have time)
2:00–2:40 Mini tour, Olive and the SAW implant, wireless biometric data
2:40–3:20 Patrick, artificial vision systems, prosthetics
3:20–4:00 Nick, artificial pancreas/diabetes, patient experience
4:00–4:20 refreshments, wrap-up

bests,
Tobie

Fig. 4.4.3

CYBORGS

—

FACT AND

FICTION?

PATRICK DEGENAAR
Lecturer in Neurobionics, Institute of Biomedical Engineering and the Division of Neuroscience, Faculty of Medicine

What are you researching?
Augmented vision. This is a method whereby we maximize the information throughput from the eye to the visual cortex by pre-filtering the visual scene and feeding this back to the patient through virtual reality headwear Optoelectronic Visual Prosthesis. For individuals whose sight has deteriorated to the extent that there is no longer any functional vision, we are investigating a revolutionary form of optoelectronic prosthesis for returning vision.

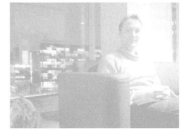

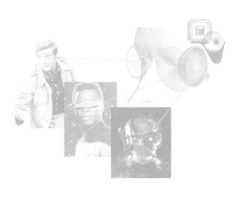

Fig. 4.4.4

4.4.3 *Extract from an email arranging interviews*
4.4.4 – 4.4.6 *Researcher profiles from information sheet interviews*

OLIVE MURPHY
Researcher, Institute of Biomedical
Engineering, Imperial College London

What are you researching?
I'm applying advanced communication technologies to mobile healthcare, in particular the high frequency design and modelling of implanted biosensors and the methodologies for interrogating implanted sensors.

An example is an implanted blood pressure sensor. Based on a tyre pressure monitor, this biosensor can be implanted without a power supply in the human body and continuously measure blood pressure. An external interrogator sends pulses of energy to activate the device, which in turns sends back a signal, which varies according to changes in blood pressure. This excites me because it applies current technology and adapts it for the benefit of mankind.

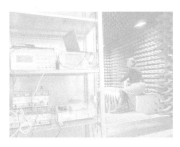

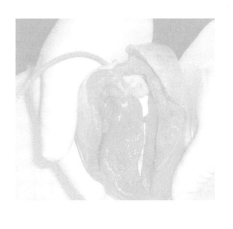

NICK OLIVER
Researcher, Institute of Biomedical
Engineering, Imperial College London.

What are you researching?
Diabetes Technology Research – A bio-inspired closed-loop insulin delivery, based on the silicon pancreatic beta-cell. I'm working on the first bio-inspired approach to glucose management of Type-I diabetic patients, using a real-time closed-loop insulin delivery system. The delivery system consists of a glucose biosensor, used with the silicon beta-cell to drive a motorised pump. Glucose-induced bursting of beta cells in the pancreas are used to control the insulin secretion in our bodies. A low-power implementation of these metabolic cells in silicon is achieved resulting in efficient glucose control.

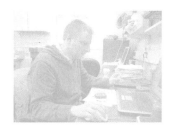

Fig. 4.4.6

Fig. 4.4.5

4·5

ON CONSTRUCTING COLLABORATIONS BETWEEN ENGINEERS, DESIGNERS AND PUBLICS

Essay by Emily Dawson
*Science and Technology Education Group, Department of Education and Professional Studies, King's College London
March 2009*

**'There are so many different ways it can, and cannot work, and I think one of the most important things is a mutual understanding of what the other person does':
On constructing collaborations between engineers, designers and publics**

To experiment with collaboration between different groups for public engagement is a challenge, as the title quote suggests. Not only is collaboration subject to multiple interpretations and expectations, but public engagement is another contested field, where aims and intentions, theories and practices are the subject of a considerable literature.[1] Material Beliefs was a multidisciplinary project that brought together designers and engineers, and sought to explore alternative models of public engagement. In total, 34 engineers and scientists, five designers and a number of members of the public were directly involved in collaborations, not to mention the much larger number of publics involved in over 40 public engagement activities. These collaborations were at the heart of the project's experiment: could collaboration between designers, engineers and publics develop innovative forms of public engagement? This essay explores the collaborative aspects of Material Beliefs, focusing on three key aspects of these collaborations: different expectations, interpersonal relationships and models of collaboration. These issues will be illustrated using quotes from the project evaluation.

Different expectations
Material Beliefs was designed to be flexible and open about what kinds of collaboration and public engagement would result from the project, thus was purposely unrestrictive about the collaborative projects it sought to nurture.

'We made our lives difficult in the end because we didn't want to describe the collaborations in projects being science art. And there are various reasons for that, but then we didn't also want to talk about it as being design for innovation and these kinds of things, because then again… you can restrict the outcome.'
DESIGNER 5

This open approach confounded the expectations of many collaborators. As might be expected given number of participants (42+), opinions differed over the degree of 'openness' inherent in the projects. The lack of defined processes and outcomes was perceived as frustrating by some and as liberating by others.

'I wasn't 100% sure what my role/relationship to Material Beliefs was. But I think there was a certain amount of let's put you together (i.e. [engineer, public, designer]) and see what happens. I found the lack of clear role – a bit disconcerting to begin with – but came to see it as being a journey of discovery. And I enjoyed the journey.'
PUBLIC 2

While designers reported being comfortable with the unrestrictive nature of Material Beliefs, within the engineering and publics collaborators, there was a split between those who embraced the lack of parameters and those who did not. Therefore differences in expectations were not driven solely by subject disciplines.

Interpersonal relationships
The second key aspect of the collaborations was the extent to which relationships were built and maintained. In two projects, a number of smaller collaborations began before the main collaboration emerged. One designer explained this informally as a process of trying to find people with whom enough mutual empathy was present for collaborative work. The degree to which collaborations were maintained was cited as criteria for success across the evaluation. Collaborators able to describe friendly interpersonal relationships reported higher levels of satisfaction, personal enjoyment and a greater perception of success for their projects. In projects where friendships were described, collaborators also went on to talk at length, via emails and informal conversations, about their plans to continue working together.

The difficulty of establishing positive collaborative relationships was also noted in the evaluation.

'I think the collaborative side of it was probably underestimated…probably most of the way through… the idea that collaboration is easy, that you can bring people together and if you don't… if you've not experienced it… it's easy you know, it's going to be successful.'
DESIGNER 3

Material Beliefs intentionally developed collaborations through a series of filmed interviews, meetings and workshops. This differs from more organic collaborations based on friendship or mutual interest and was highlighted by a range of participants across the evaluation. Projects where collaborators were able to develop friendlier relationships also developed a 'co-production' model of communication, while those where interpersonal relationships were less established tended to describe their projects in terms of a 'one-sided' model of collaboration.

Models of collaboration: One-sided collaboration
Two collaborative models can be distinguished among the projects. In the first model, collaborations tended to be one-sided, guided predominantly by one discipline, which 'used' the other (see Fig. 4.5.1). This model appeared in more than one project and at different times within projects. This model was described by both engineers and designers, and at different points either engineering or design was portrayed as the dominant force of a project.

'I mean, the idea for these [objects] came completely from [the designers], there was no engineering input on those whatsoever. It's kind of we gave birth to the idea, pretty much defined the [objects], [an engineer] helped with that a little bit, but this is why for me the collaborative side of it failed because the idea came solely from the design side, the engineering came in, [a second engineer] was fantastic but he came in so late that we already had pretty much outlined [the objects] fairly well.'
DESIGNER 2

This model of collaboration appeared in projects where collaborators seemed to have little sense of what the design role was and attached only limited value to it.

'[He] said, "I'm not an artist. I'm a designer." And something that interested me is always, how do you... what does a designer do that the artist doesn't? For example, is it like an architect and a civil engineer, where the architect does the fluff and the engineer makes it happen.'
ENGINEER 9

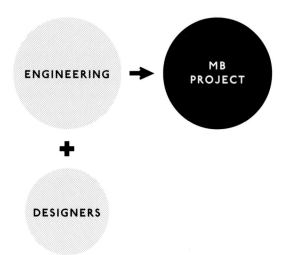

Fig. 4.5.1 *One-sided model of collaboration*

In a symmetrical manner, some designers described difficulties communicating clearly about their work, their role in the project and, in particular, the differences between various aspects of design – for example, between product design and speculative/critical design.

'And you see it all over the TV, Linda Baker and celebrity designers working for MFI and if that's what they think they're getting then... it's difficult for us to get a foot in the door because all they think that we're doing, is to be maybe take their sort of, wonderfully engineered things and... package it in pretty ways. And if that's what they think then of course it's problematic...'
DESIGNER 2

Misconceptions about the role played by designers, and frustration with the open nature of the whole project – both tended to occur in collaborations which were relatively one-sided, and which also exhibited more formality in their approach to interpersonal relationships.

Collaboration as co-production
In the second model, both disciplines worked together to 'co-produce' a project for public engagement. This involved more emphasis on working with publics and a greater degree of relationship building (see Fig. 4.5.2). In this model, collaboration was characterised by an acceptance of undefined roles and an appreciation that the project outcomes were open and therefore unknown.

'I didn't mind not having a clear goal... I quite enjoyed, in fact, not having one because everything else we do does have one so it's quite nice, it's, rather than thinking, "Right if I do this I must make sure that I measure that at the end and I must have these criteria for that measurement. Whereas, you know, just have a chat. Fine. And, and that's, that's liberating personally.'"
ENGINEER 15

One of the groups that developed this model in their collaboration were also able to involve members of the public directly in their project. This may be because practices common to some forms of public engagement have been developing similarly open, participatory approaches to engagement.

In the co-production model, collaborators not only embraced the open nature of Material Beliefs, but described confusion about roles or misunderstandings about design in neutral or positive terms.

> 'I think previously, the Venn diagrams of sort of the languages that we use and, and the skill sets that we had, would have been miles apart and they sort of gradually come together and now there is this sort of overlap where we speak the same language and, and have similar ways of thinking... And for me it's mostly been changing the boundaries that we use to describe things... so I don't think that it's been quite that straightforward and some people have been much more scientific and some people have been much more artistic. But it, it's been about flexibility of language and ways of thinking and, and thinking differently about problems and learning not to think in the box of feasibility which is what you're saying isn't it? Stop thinking about what's credible and think about what, what might be incredible.'
> ENGINEER 13

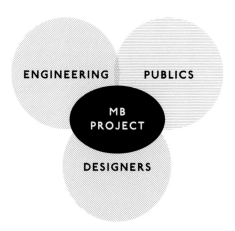

Fig. 4.5.2 *Co-production model of collaboration*

This description of the 'incredible' contrasts with the negative associations developed about confusion over the role of design, frustration at the lack of clear management in the project and a tendency towards 'one-sided' models of collaboration. Being flexible about positioning designers, engineers and publics in relation to one another and the capacity to embrace the open ended nature of Material Beliefs may be connected to the ability of a collaborative project to develop a 'co-production' model of collaboration.

Conclusions

This essay has illustrated the three key collaborative themes that emerged from the Material Beliefs evaluation: how collaborators managed the open-ended nature of the project, the impact of friendly relationships, and the two models of collaboration that developed across the projects. These issues have been referred to as the tensions between 'collaborative advantage' and 'collaborative inertia' (Huxham and Vagen, 2005). 'Collaborative advantage' describes how working together provides collaborators with access to knowledge and skills beyond those held individually, opening numerous opportunities for strategic collaborations. 'Collaborative inertia' concerns the frustrations, mismatch of expectations, and frequent failures of seemingly exciting collaborations to achieve their potential, caused by problems in communication, management and relations (Huxham and Vagen, 2005).

Constructing collaborations between different disciplines is a complicated and nuanced practice. Material Beliefs can be best understood as an umbrella project that created a space for collaborators to develop new relationships and novel forms of working, and to expand their public engagement practices. 'One-sided' and 'co-production' models of collaboration are appropriate, in varying degrees, depending on the context and nature of a project. What is interesting in this project is the extent to which other factors (interpersonal relationships and degree of comfort with the open ended nature of the projects) cluster around a particular model and suggest underlying tensions in the 'one-sided' model.

While constructed collaborations may always differ from more organic partnerships, the processes involved deserve reflection and further experimentation. In particular, the issues of managing relationships, balancing collaborators' needs, communication and the different models of collaboration should be considered further in light of this project.

1 In the last 30 years a range of communication techniques have developed around science, designed to better manage the public's perceptions of science as well as relationships between science, government, industry and public's (Bauer and Gregory 2007, Gregory et al 2007). One development in this field has been the 'public understanding of science' (PUS) movement, which has more recently evolved into 'public engagement with science and technology' (PEST) (Irwin and Wynne 1996, Miller 2001). PEST practices were intended to attempt to redress the balance between science, publics and broader socio-political concerns (House of Lords 2000, Wynne 2007).

Reference List

Bauer M. W. and Gregory J. 2007. 'From journalism to corporate communication in post-war Britain'. Pp. 33 – 51. In Bauer M.W. and Bucchi M. (eds.). *Journalism, Science and Society*. New York and Abingdon: Routledge.

Gregory J. Agar J. Lock S. and Harris S. 2007. 'Public engagement of science in the private sector: A new form of PR?'. Pp. 203-214. In Bauer M.W. and Bucchi M. (eds.). *Journalism, Science and Society*. New York and Abingdon: Routledge.

House of Lords. 2000. *Science in Society*. London: Her Majesty's Stationary Office. www.publications. parliament.uk/pa/ld199900/ldselect/ldsctech/38/3801.htm accessed 9.11.08.

Huxham C. and Vagen S. 2005. *Managing to collaborate. The theory and practice of collaborative advantage*. Abingdon and New York; Routledge.

Irwin A. and Wynne B. 1996. 'Introduction'. Pp.1-18 in *Misunderstanding Science? The public reconstruction of science and technology*. Irwin A. and Wynne B. (eds.). Cambridge: Cambridge University Press.

Miller S. 2001. 'Public understanding of science at the crossroads". *Public Understanding of Science*. 10: 115-120.

Wynne B. 2006. 'Public engagement as a Means of Restoring Public Trust in Science – Hitting the Notes, but Missing the Music'. *Community Genetics*. 9: 211-220.

Colour Plates

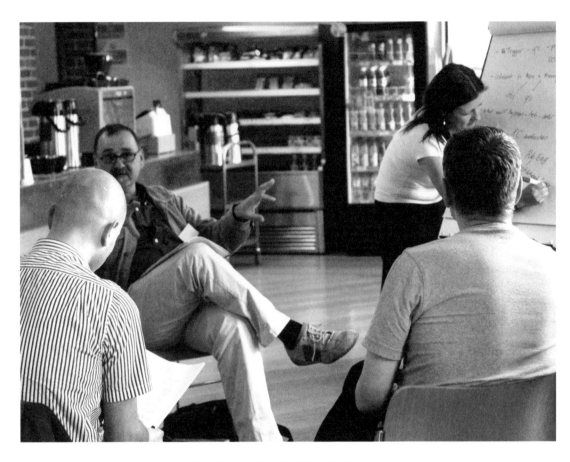

Fig. 5.1 *Brainstorming at the Collaboration Workshop*

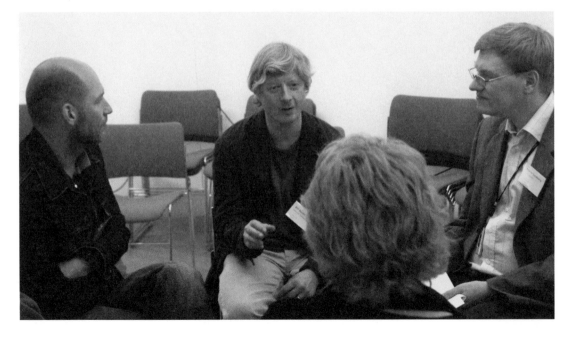

Fig. 5.2 *Jimmy, Bill, Karen and Anders in conversation at the Collaboration Workshop*

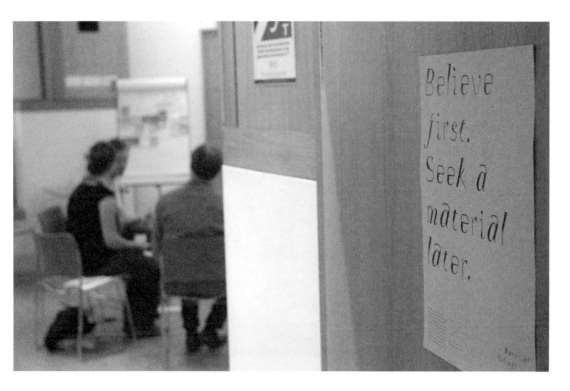

Fig. 5.3 *A comment from a workshop attendee displayed as a poster*

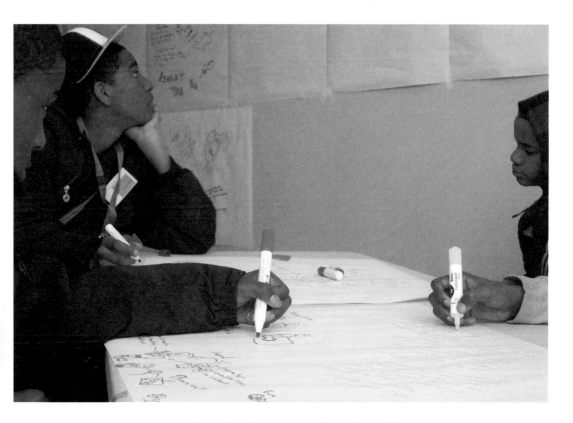

Fig. 5.4 *Students at the Stephen Lawrence Centre discuss cyborgs and robots*

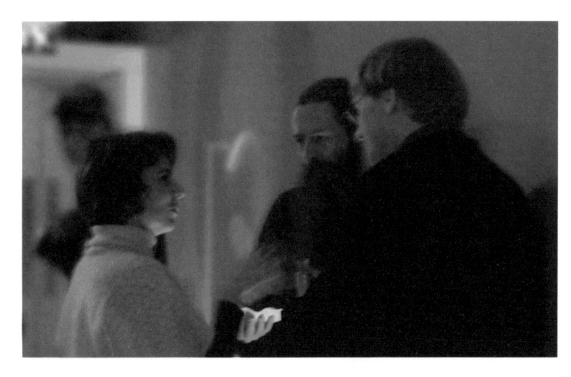

Fig. 5.5 *Susana, Aubrey and Anders at the Dana Centre*

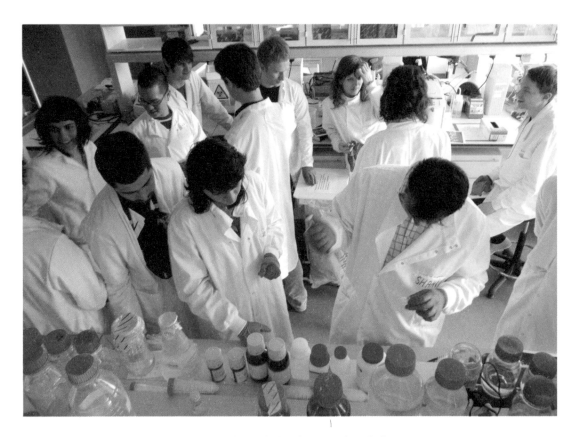

Fig. 5.6 *Extracting DNA from cheek cells at the Institute of Biomedical Engineering*

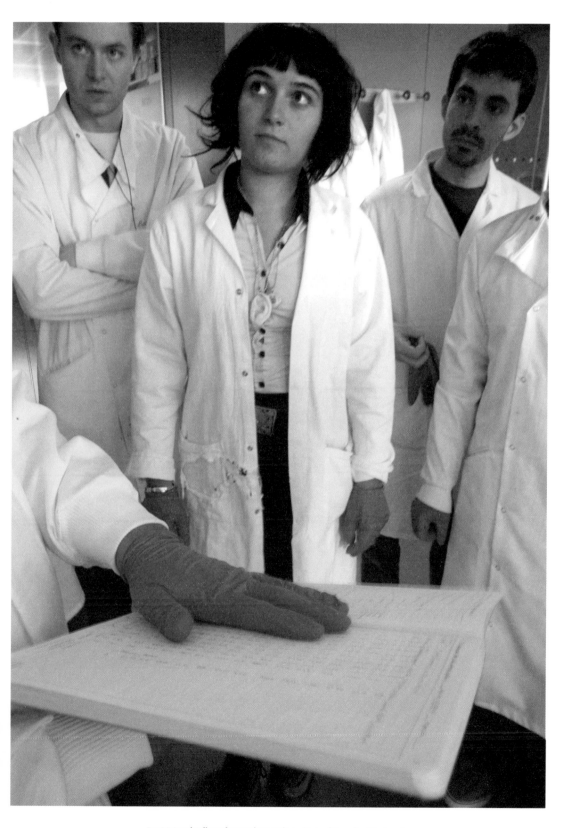

Fig. 5.7 *Royal College of Art students at the Institute of Biomedical Engineering*

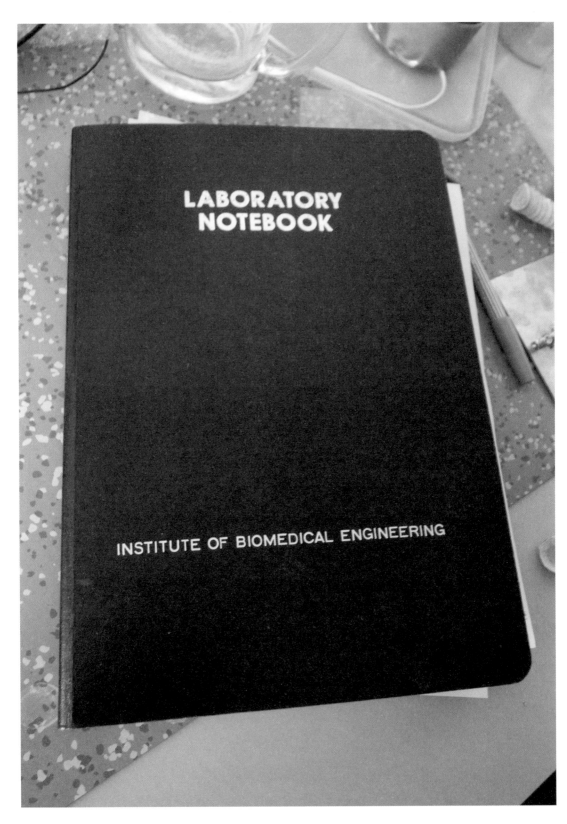

Fig. 5.8 *Laboratory notebooks can be identified by a unique number on the spine*

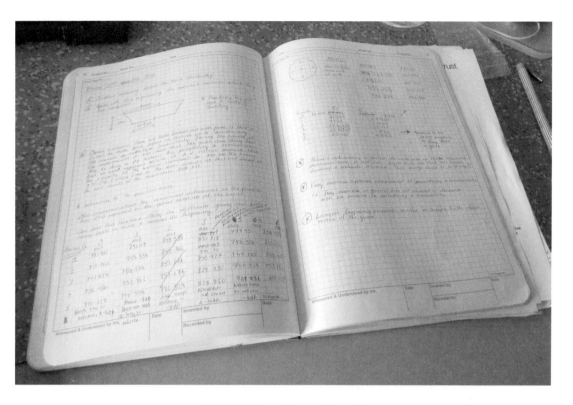

Fig. 5.9 *Notebooks provide a record of research*

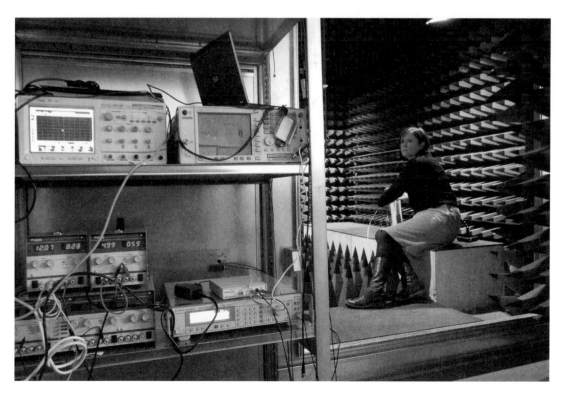

Fig. 5.10 *Olive tests the performance of an implantable blood pressure monitor*

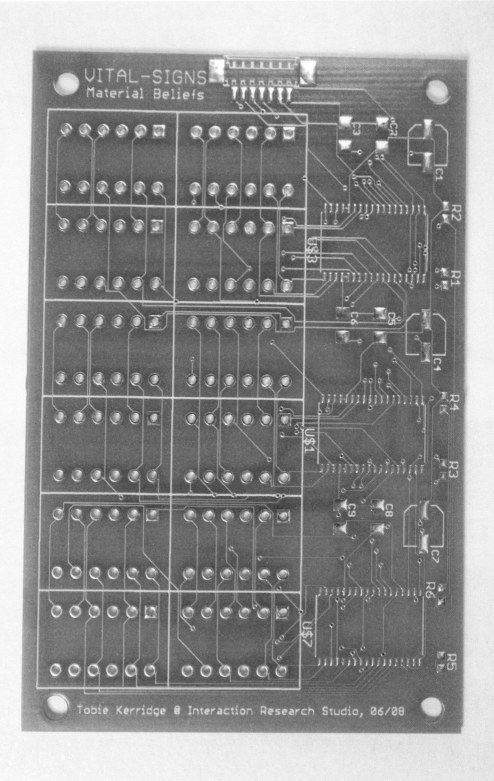

Fig. 5.11 *A printed circuit board manufactured for a prototype*

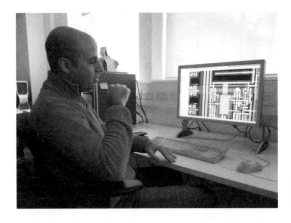

Fig. 5.12 *Tim describes software he used to design silicon chips*

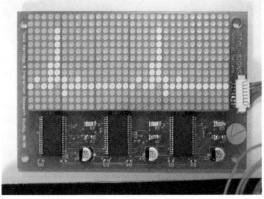

Fig. 5.13 *A printed circuit board with components soldered into place*

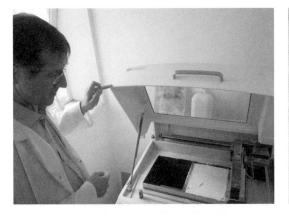

Fig. 5.14 *Cases being printed using a rapid prototyping machine*

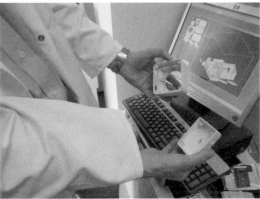

Fig. 5.15 *Printed parts shown alongside CAD models*

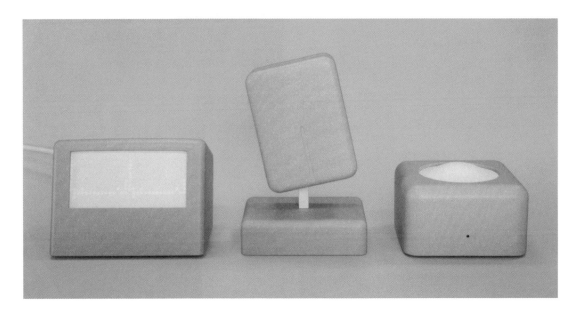

Fig. 5.16 *Finished Vital Signs prototypes*

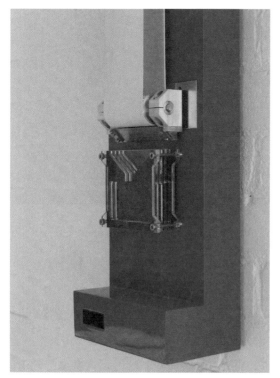

Fig. 5.17 *Flypaper Robotic Clock*

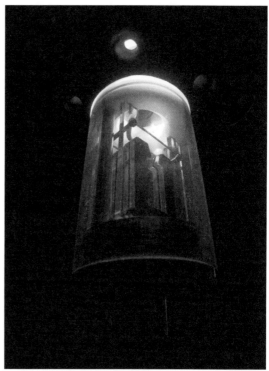

Fig. 5.18 *Lampshade Robot*

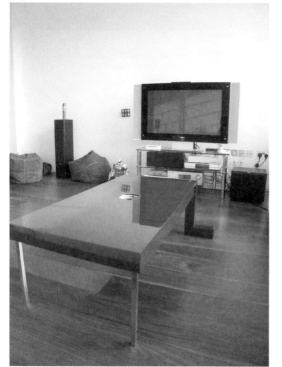

Fig. 5.19 *Coffee Table Mousetrap Robot*

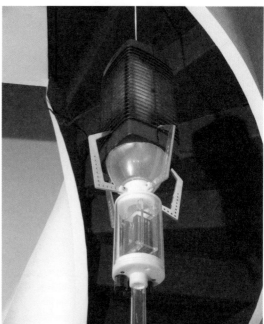

Fig. 5.20 *UV Fly Killer Parasite*

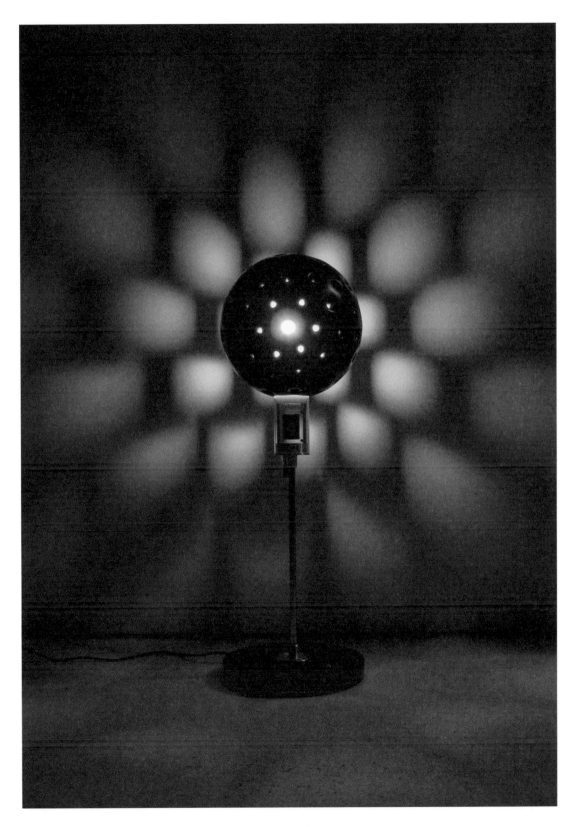

Fig. 5.21 *Lampshade Robot*

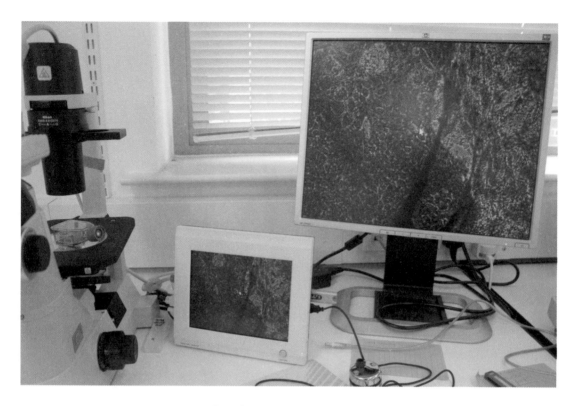

Fig. 5.22 *Colonies of stained stem cells viewed through a microscope*

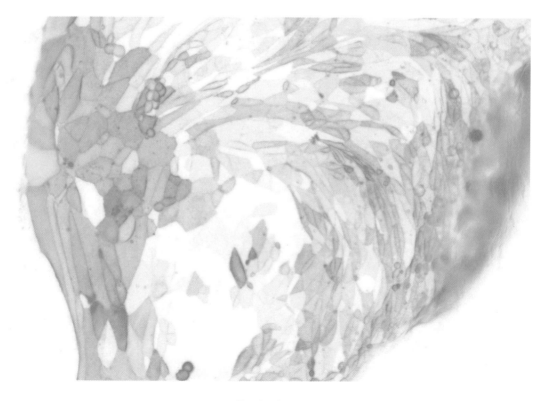

Fig. 5.23 *Human stem cells in the early stages of differentiation*

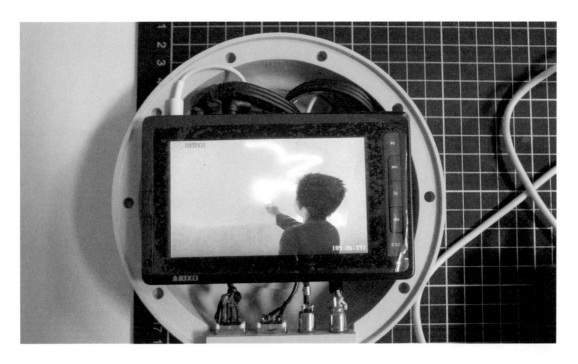

Fig. 5.24 *The Neuroscope fitted with screen*

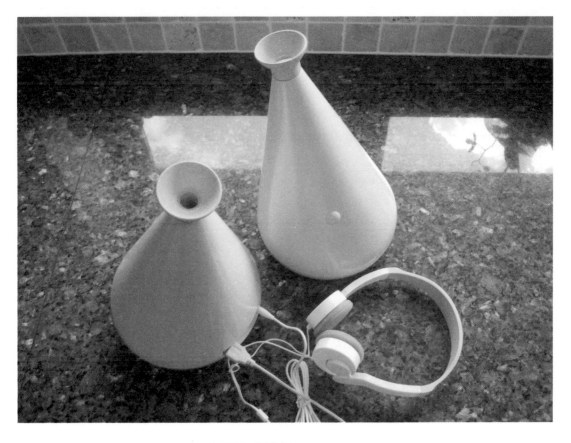

Fig. 5.25 *Two finished Neuroscope prototypes*

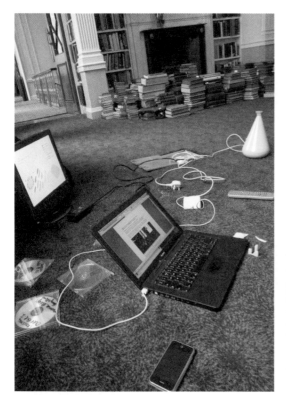

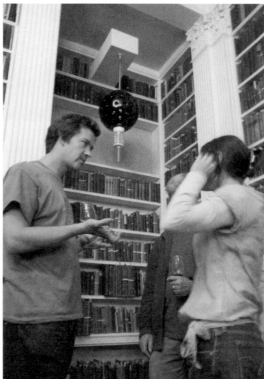

Fig. 5.26 *Installing work at the Royal Institution*   Fig. 5.27 *Royal Institution exhibition opening*

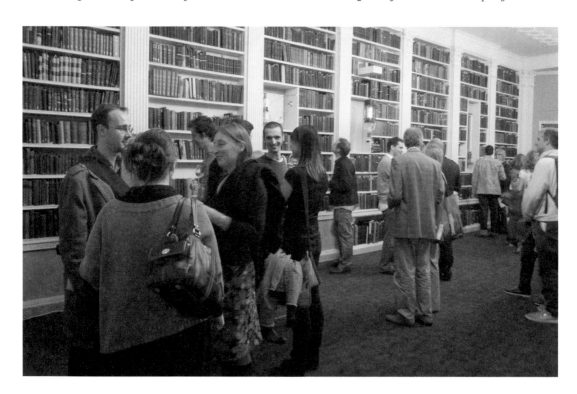

Fig. 5.28 *Royal Institution exhibition opening*

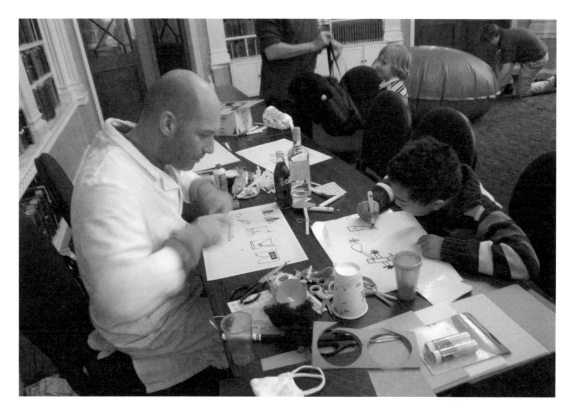

Fig. 5.29 *Designing fly-eating robots at the Royal Institution*

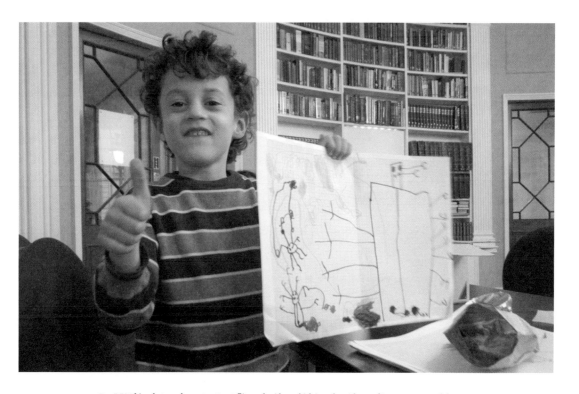

Fig. 5.30 *This robot uses honey to attract flies and spiders which it grabs with one of its many arms and then eats*

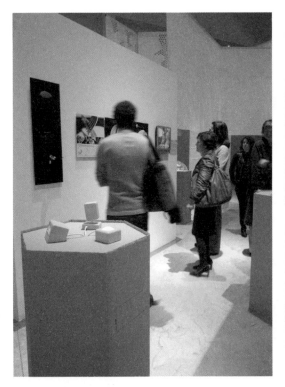

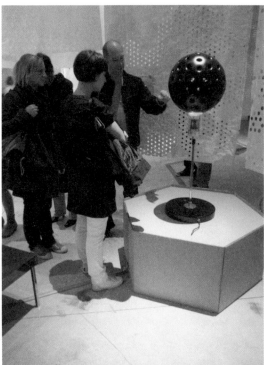

Fig. 5.32 *Nowhere/Now/Here exhibition opening*　　　　　Fig. 5.33 *Nowhere/Now/Here exhibition opening*

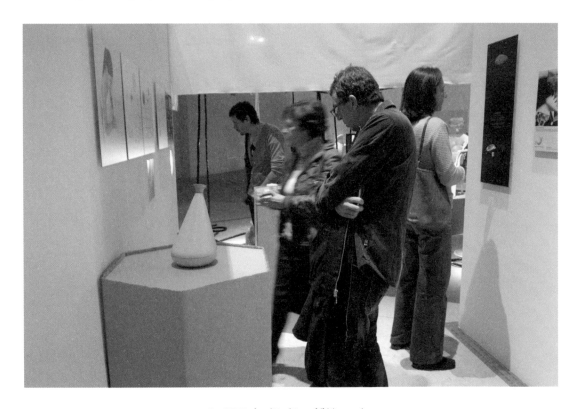

Fig. 5.31 *Nowhere/Now/Here exhibition opening*

Appendices

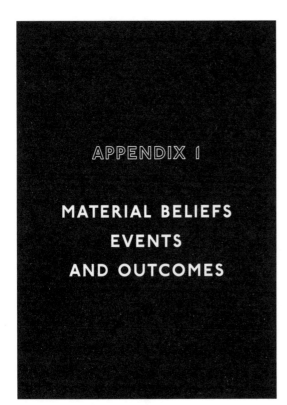

APPENDIX I

MATERIAL BELIEFS
EVENTS
AND OUTCOMES

10 August – 27 October 2007
Our Cyborg Future
Discovery Museum, Blandford Square, Newcastle upon Tyne
NE1 4JA, UK
The exhibition was part of the DOTT festival in Newcastle.
Material Beliefs exhibited existing work from the
Biojewellery project, and offered new relationships and
alliances with scientists, designers, and artists.
www.dott07.com/go/health/our-cyborg-future-me-or-machine

15 October 2007
Junior Scientifique
Thomas Hepburn School, Swards Road, Felling, Gateshead,
Tyne and Wear NE10 9UZ, UK
An after school club in Gateshead invited members from
Material Beliefs to present and discuss their work. Ten year
8 students attended and provided thoughtful feedback on
cybernetic eyes and tissue engineering.
www.juniorcafesci.org.uk

15 October 2007
Café Culture / Café Scientifique – Our Future
Human Body?
World Headquarters, Curtis Mayfield House, Carliol Square,
Newcastle upon Tyne NE1 6UF, UK
An evening Café Scientifique in Newcastle, Material Beliefs
appeared alongside other researchers working in the field
of cybernetics. With an audience of about twenty-five, this
was an event that encouraged discussion on technology and
body ability, and demonstrated how technology provokes
controversy amongst particular groups of users when it
becomes situated in society.
www.cafescientifique.org/newcastle.htm

29 October – 2 November 2007
TU/e Industrial Design Masters course, Eindhoven,
Netherlands
TU/e, Den Dolech 2, 5612 AZ Eindhoven, Netherlands
A two-day workshop for masters students in the faculty of
Industrial Design at Technische Universiteit Eindhoven.
Methods that had evolved from the process of setting
up collaboration between designers and engineers were
deployed in this workshop, which encourages students
to interview researchers in their university, and develop
a debate, discussion of design scenario from unexpected
findings.
w3.tue.nl/en

22 January 2008
Techno Bodies; Hybrid Life?
The Dana Centre,165 Queen's Gate, South Kensington, London
SW7 5HD, UK
An evening of debate at Science Museum's Dana Centre,
focused on Material Beliefs emerging themes. Each of the
four project clusters curated an area of discussion, and each
area had it's own invited speakers.
www.danacentre.org.uk/events/2008/01/22/354

24 January 2008
EPSRC PPE Award workshop
The Dana Centre,165 Queen's Gate, South Kensington, London SW7 5HD, UK
An information day for scientists, engineers and project partners who are interested in applying for EPSRC Partnership for Public Engagement grants. Material Beliefs was invited to this event to present Biojewellery, as a PPE case study.
www.the-ba.net/the-ba/ScienceinSociety/EPSRC_workshops

6 – 9 February 2008
Swiss STS Meeting 2008 – ScienceFutures
Universität Zürich / ETH, Rämistrasse 64, CH-8001 Zürich, Switzerland
An academic event where Material Beliefs was presented as supporting studies by two PhD candidates. This was also a networking event for the project, within a broad and vibrant community of young European researchers .
www.zgw.ethz.ch/sts

1 March 2008
Design and the Elastic Mind
The Museum of Modern Art, 11 West 53 Street, New York, NY 10019-5497, USA
A presentation and a discussion with sociologists, design and art students. Part of the events programme supporting the Design and the Elastic Mind exhibition.
www.moma.org/exhibitions/exhibitions.php?id=5632

14 March 2008
New Sciences of Protection – Designing safe living
IAS Building, County South, Lancaster University, Lancaster LA1 4YD, UK
A Presentation and a workshop for researchers, sociologists, designers and students.
www.lancs.ac.uk/ias/annualprogramme/protection/conference/index.htm

18 March – 1 April May 2008
Talking with Experts
College of Visual and Performing Arts, Syracuse University, Syracuse, NY 13244-1010, USA
A presentation of Material Beliefs methods and outcomes, followed by a discussion and workshop with design students, researchers and scientists.
www.vpa.syr.edu

19 March 2008
Mind the Loop
Institute for Biomedical Engineering, Imperial College London, South Kensington Campus, London SW7 2AZ, UK
A filmed conversation between an engineer, a patient, a doctor and a designer, to discuss emerging technologies for the treatment of diabetes.
www.materialbeliefs.com/events/loop.php

2 – 3 April 2008
ISDN3 – Material Beliefs; Technology for People
School of Design, City Campus East, Newcastle upon Tyne NE1 8ST, UK
An doctoral research event where Material Beliefs was presented to a community of researchers. Presentations focused on the design of services for a range of user groups, and the forty attendees were from design and public service backgrounds.
www.northumbria.ac.uk/sd/academic/scd/whatson/news/listen/808653

8 – 10 April 2008
Ignite – My Space, My City, My World
The Stephen Lawrence Centre, 39 Brookmill Road, London SE8 4HU, UK
Material Beliefs was invited to lead workshops on two days of this three-day conference for year 10 students. This was held at the new Steven Lawrence Centre in Deptford. The conference was designed to 'build young people's confidence in making their voices heard in the places where decisions are made about design, engineering, economics and the future.'
www.ignitefutures.org.uk/ignite-projects/steven-lawrence

18 – 19 April 2008
Design and the Elastic Mind – Science teachers inset day
Museum of Modern Art, 11 W 53rd St New York, NY 10019, USA
Presentation and discussion with teachers from science and art disciplines.

21 – 22 April 2008
Material beliefs Workshop – IBE and Design Interactions, RCA London
Institute for Biomedical Engineering, Imperial College London, South Kensington Campus, London SW7 2AZ, UK
Students and staff at the Design Interactions course at the Royal College of Art took part in a two day workshop at the Institute of Biomedical Engineering. The aim of the workshop was to provide those from the RCA with an embedded view upon biomedical technologies, and for those based at IBE to have a refreshed set of responses to their research.
www.materialbeliefs.com/events/rca-ibe.php

30 April 2008
Material Beliefs – evening lecture
Central Saint Martins College of Art and Design, Southampton Row, London WC1B 4AP, UK
A presentation followed by discussion with undergraduate design students.

14 May 2008
Disruptive design
General Electrics Healthcare, Waukesha, Chicago, USA
The workshop explored the premise that by demonstrating that a research proposal could identify and consult with a range of stakeholders, the quality of the proposal would be improved, and more likely to secure funding.

23 May 2008
Design Blast Conference
Karlsruhe University of Art and Design, Karlsruhe, Germany
A presentation and discussion with design students, academics, practitioners and the public.
designblast.hfg-karlsruhe.de

16 & 23 May 2008
Science and Society – IBE and Design Interactions, RCA London
Design Interactions, Royal College of Art, Kensington Gore, London SW7 2EU, UK
A project for Design Interactions students, with researchers at IBE and Reading taking up visiting tutor roles at the RCA through tutorial sessions.
www.materialbeliefs.com/events/rca-ibe.php

14 July 2008
Selfridges & Co – Wonder Wall
Ground floor, Selfridges London, 400 Oxford St, London W1A 1AB, UK
Biojewellery is included in *Natural History*, an exhibition installed at the Wonder Wall, a temporary exhibition in the Wonder Room on the ground floor of Selfridges, London.
www.thewonderroom.selfridges.com

24 – 27 July 2008
Secret Garden Party Festival
Guerilla Science tent, Secret Garden Party, Huntingdon near Cambridge, UK
Part of a programme of tented science demonstrations, our session explores how bodies and products become connected through new technologies. Some initial slides showed images of everyday hybrids including gamers and karaoke singers.
www.materialbeliefs.com/events/sgp.php

31 July 2008
Bioengineering public interviews – Selfridges Wonder Room
Ground floor, Selfridges London, 400 Oxford St, London W1A 1AB, UK
A series of filmed conversations with shoppers at Selfridges about the value of collaborations between speculative design and biomedical engineering, based at the *Natural History* exhibition.
www.thewonderroom.selfridges.com

4 September 2008
9th World Congress of Bioethics
Rijeka, Croatia
A paper was presented at this academic event, organised by the International Association of Bioethics, under the patronage of UNESCO.
www.bioethicsworldcongress.com

12 September 2008
The Future Object 2008
V&A South Kensington, Cromwell Road, London SW7 2RL, UK
V&A ThinkTanks – a public think tank on the future of designed objects, based in the new Sackler Centre for arts education.
www.vam.ac.uk/school_stdnts/education_centre/index.html

19 September 2008
24 hr design and make
121-123 Deptford High Street, Deptford, London SE8 4NS, UK
An attempt to demonstrate what can be created in 24 hours. Starting at 7a.m. a number of teams will be provided with basic materials, tools and a brief to bring together objects, drawings, illustrations, installation, sound, video, and textiles.
www.24hrdesignandmake.co.uk

19 September 2008
This Happened
Design Museum, Shad Thames, London SE1 2YD, UK
This Happened is a series of events focusing on the stories behind interaction design. Tobie Kerridge, Yuri Suzuki and Cinimod Studio presented projects at the Design Museum.
www.thishappened.org/archive/sep-2008

1 October – 21 November 2008
Crossing Over
The Royal Institution of Great Britain, 21 Albemarle Street, London W1S 4BS, UK
Art, design and science combine to address bioengineering. This exhibition in the newly renovated building includes work from all four of the Material Beliefs collaborations.
www.crossingover-exhibition.co.uk

7 October 2008 – 21 November 2008
Nowhere/Now/Here
LABoral Centro de Arte y Creación Industrial, Los Prados, 121 – 33394 Gijon, Spain
Nowhere/Now/Here is a major exhibition exploring the world of objects we decide to surround ourselves with.
www.laboralcentrodearte.org/exhibitions/show/77

14 October 2008

Arts & Technology: The Role of the Arts in Democratic Policy Making

National Theatre, South Bank, London SE1 9PX, UK

When it comes to developments in science and technology, public perceptions on these issues are influenced largely by the various sources in the public square including the media and the arts.

www.bioethics.ac.uk/index.php?do=events&rid=164

22 October 2008

Crossing over: fusing science and art

The Royal Institution of Great Britain, 21 Albemarle Street, London W1S 4BS, UK

Mark Lythgoe facilitates a discussion about how artists and scientists have each inspired each other to look at their work in a different light.

www.rigb.org/contentControl?action=displayContent& id=00000002278

28 October 2008

BioPlay

The Dana Centre, 165 Queen's Gate, South Kensington, London SW7 5HD, UK

Explore how brain cells are being fused with interactive devices, and discover kits that are harvesting and banking body cells.

www.danacentre.org.uk/events/2008/10

28 October 2008

ESRC Genomics & Society

Savoy Place, 2 Savoy Place, London WC2R 0BL, UK

A poster presenting the collaborations and project outcomes of Material Beliefs

www.genomicsandsociety.org

1 November 2008

Family fun day

The Royal Institution of Great Britain, 21 Albemarle Street, London W1S 4BS, UK

Design and make your own fly eating robot with the help of Dr Weeble and Dr Fly. With a microbial fuel cell as it's stomach, your robot can generate energy from fly juice to power your toys.

www.rigb.org/contentControl?action=displayContent& id=2358

8 & 11 November 2008

Cyborgs and Hybrids

Roundhouse, Chalk Farm Road, London NW1 8EH, UK

LIVE TV! is a ten week course for young people run by tutors at Camden's Roundhouse, resulting in 4 live TV shows. One show explores the fact and fiction of Cyborgs. A group interviewed researchers about biomedical implants.

www.roundhouse.org.uk/about

24 November 2008

Sci-Art Film

Institute for Biomedical Engineering, Imperial College London, South Kensington Campus, London SW7 2AZ, UK

Interviews by Richard Wylie from Science TV about the relationship between the two cultures of science and design.

19 – 23 December 2008

Touch Me Festival

Student Centre, Zagreb, Croatia

Organized by KONTEJNER, Bureau of Contemporary Arts Practice, the Touch Me festival focuses on art at the intersection of emergent technology.

www.touchme-festival.org

28 – 29 January 2009

Interactivos?09: Garage Science

Medialab Prado, Plaza de las Letras. C/ Alameda, 15 · 28014 Madrid, Spain

An International Workshop-Seminar that includes an intensive project development workshop and a seminar with lectures and public theoretical works presentations.

medialab-prado.es/article/taller-seminario_interactivos09 _ciencia_de_garaje

16 – 18 February 2009

Tangible and Embedded Interaction 2009

University Arms Hotel, Regent Street, Cambridge, Cambridgeshire CB2 1AD, UK

An academic paper at TEI09.

www.tei-conf.org/index.html

20 February 2009

Is Design Good for You?

University of Brighton, 57-68 Grand Parade, Brighton BN2 2JY, UK

A symposium exploring interdisciplinary approaches to learning and teaching in art, design and health in Higher Education. In association with The Centre for Excellence in Teaching and Learning through Design and The Higher Education Academy Subject Centres in Health Sciences & Practice, and Art, Design, Media.

cetld.brighton.ac.uk/events/is-design-good-for-you

27 February – 2 March 2009

Kinetica Artfair 2009

P3, University of Westminster, 35 Marylebone Road, London NW1 5LS, UK

Kinetica Art Fair is dedicated to kinetic, robotic, sound, light and time-based art.

www.kinetica-artfair.com

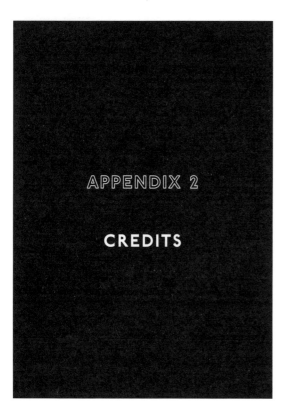

APPENDIX 2

CREDITS

PICTURE CREDITS

Photographs, illustrations and film stills are owned by the following contributors.

Every effort has been made to trace the copyright holders of the visual material reproduced in this publication. The publishers and editors apologise to anyone who has not been reached.

JULIEN ANDERSON 1.5.2 – 1.5.6, 5.1 – 5.3
JAMES AUGER, JIMMY LOIZEAU
& ALEKSANDAR ZIVANOVIC 3.3.19 – 3.3.35, 5.17 – 5.21
NELLY BEN HAYOUN 2.3.14, 2.3.15
ELIO CACCAVALE 1.6.1, 1.6.3 – 1.6.5, 1.6.7 – 1.6.10,
3.5.11, 3.5.12, 3.5.14 – 3.5.19, 3.5.23 – 3.5.28, 3.5.39 – 3.5.41,
5.24, 5.25
WILL CAREY 2.3.16
CHANNEL 4 NEWS 4.1.9
EMILY CULME-SEYMOUR 5.23
REVITAL COHEN 3.2.27
TIM CONSTANDINOU 3.2.5
JULIE DANIELS 3.4.8 – 3.4.11, 3.4.15, 3.4.16
EMILY DAWSON 4.5.1, 4.5.2
PATRICK DEGANAAR 4.4.4
DAISY GINSBERG 2.3.17
JOHN GREENMAN, IOANNIS IEROPOULOS
& CHRIS MELHUISH 3.3.2 – 3.3.4
MARK HAMMOND 2.1.7 – 2.1.12, 3.5.2 – 3.5.9, 3.5.22, 5.4
HYPERKIT 1.4.1 – 1.4.5, 1.5.1
STEVE JACKMAN 2.1.3, 2.1.4, 2.1.16, 2.2.7 – 2.2.10, 2.3.7,
3.2.16, 3.3.18, 3.4.1, 3.4.12, 3.5.1, 3.5.10, 3.5.29, 4.2.27
TOBIE KERRIDGE 0.1 – 0.5, 1.1.3 – 1.1.6, 1.6.5,
1.6.7 – 1.6.11, 1.6.13, 1.6.14, 2.1.1, 2.1.2, 2.1.13, 2.1.14,
2.1.16, 2.1.17, 2.3.2 – 2.3.6, 3.2.1, 3.2.2, 3.2.4, 3.2.6,
3.2.8 – 3.2.11, 3.2.13, 3.2.17 – 3.2.26, 3.3.1, 4.1.1 – 4.1.3,
4.2.1 – 4.2.6, 4.2.9, 4.2.10, 4.2.12 – 4.2.15, 4.3.3 – 4.3.5,
4.3.8, 4.3.9, 4.3.12 – 4.3.14, 4.4.1, 5.6 – 5.16, 5.26 – 5.30
TOBIE KERRIDGE, NIKKI STOTT & IAN THOMPSON
1.1.1, 1.1.2
CATHRINE KRAMER 2.3.12, 2.3.13
JIMMY LOIZEAU 3.3.1, 3.3.14 – 3.3.17
VEDRAN METELKO & KONTEJNER 4.1.5, 4.1.7 – 4.1.9
OLIVE MURPHY 3.2.3, 4.4.5
DAVID MUTH 3.5.30 – 3.5.38
NICK OLIVER 3.2.7, 4.4.6
SASCHA POHFLEPP 2.3.10, 2.3.11
PRINCESS PRODUCTIONS FOR CUTTING EDGE 3.2.12
ANDY ROBINSON 2.2.1, 2.2.3 – 2.2.6, 5.5
SUSANA SOARES 1.6.15, 1.6.17, 1.6.18, 2.1.15, 2.1.18,
3.4.2 – 3.4.7, 3.4.13, 3.4.14, 3.4.17 – 3.4.23, 5.23v
PAUL SOUTH 3.5.20, 3.5.21
ROBIN JAMES TURNER 3.5.42 – 3.5.44
VARIOUS; INTERNET IMAGE SEARCH 3.2.14, 3.2.15,
3.3.5 – 3.3.13
VARIOUS; YOUNG DESIGNERS 4.2.8, 4.2.11, 4.2.16
DIMITRIS XYDAS 3.5.13

TEXT CREDITS

1.2.1 House of Lords, Select Committee on Science and Technology, Third Report: 'Science and Society', 23 February 2000

1.2.2 Engineering Ideas in Public Engagement: Call for Participants, EPSRC, 2006

1.2.3 Reporter, the newspaper of Imperial College London, Issue 190, 17th April 2008

1.3.1, 1.3.2 Standard Proposal, 'Material Beliefs: Collaborations for Public Engagement Between Engineers and Designers', EPSRC reference EP/E035051/1, submitted 11/08/2006

1.6.2 D. Xydas, D. Norcott, K. Warwick, B. Whalley, S. Nasuto, V. Becerra, M. Hammond, J. Downes, and S. Marshall, 'Architecture for Neuronal Cell Control of a Mobile Robot', Springer Tracts in Advanced Robotics, vol. 44, pp. 23-31, 2008

1.6.6 Toumazou, C. and C. Y. Lee (2005). 'Ultra-low power UWB for real time biomedical wireless sensing.' Proceedings of the IEEE International Symposium on Circuits and Systems 1:4

1.6.12 Ieropoulos, I., Greenman, J. and Melhuish, C. (2003), 'Imitating Metabolism: Energy Autonomy in Biologically Inspired Robotics', In Proceedings of the AISB '03, Second International Symposium on Imitation in Animals and Artifacts: 191-194

1.6.18 Mason C. and Dunnill P. A brief definition of regenerative medicine. Regenerative Medicine. 3(1), 1-5, 2008

2.3.8, 2.3.9 Miah, A. (2008). Human futures : art in an age of uncertainty. Liverpool, Liverpool University Press

2.2.2, 4.1.4 Dana Centre webpages, www.danacentre.org.uk/events/2008/01/22/354 & www.danacentre.org.uk/events/2008/10/28/446, accessed on 12/2/09

4.1.5 Bago, I., et al. (2009), Touch Me Festival: Feel Better. Zagreb, KONTEJNER

4.3.1, 4.3.2 Nowhere/Now/Here exhibition invitation, 26/9/08

4.3.6, 4.3.7, 4.3.10, 4.3.11 Feo, R. and Hurtado, R. (2008). Nowhere/Now/Here. Gijón LABoral Centro de Arte y Creación Industrial

4.2.17 Royal Institution of Great Britian webpage, www.rigb.org/contentControl?action=displayContent&id=2358, accessed on 108/1/09

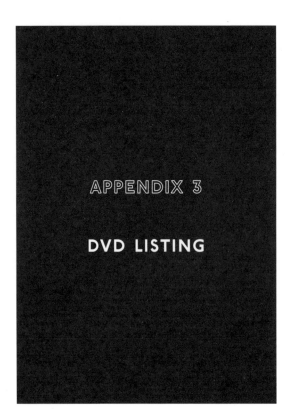

APPENDIX 3

DVD LISTING

Stills from films shot and edited by Steve Jackman appear throughout the book. The 18 films were produced to document key Material Beliefs events, and are included on the DVD.

1 **Junior Scientifique – Bionic vision** 07:59
2 **Junior Scientifique – Biojewellery** 05:15
3 **Cyborgs at Newcastle Café Scientifique** 15:56
4 **Julian Vincent interview** 11:12
5 **Neuroscope meeting at the University of Reading** 07:08
6 **Aubrey de Grey interview** 11:02
7 **Anders Sandberg interview** 07:22
8 **Techno Bodies; Hybrid Life? at the Dana Centre** 20:22
9 **Managing type 1 diabetes** 04:51
10 **A silicon pancreas** 02:52
11 **Type 1 diabetes discussion** 13:18
12 **Vital Signs description** 03:30
13 **CDER description** 12:08
14 **Interviewing shoppers at Selfridges** 03:57
15 **Neuroscope description** 04:57
16 **Bonsai Cells description** 04:49
17 **Royal College of Art tutorial** 15:20
18 **Family day at the Royal Institution** 03:27